THE MISSING HALF OF YOUR BLOOD TEST

WHY TIMING, CONTEXT, AND PATTERN MATTER MORE THAN A SINGLE NUMBER

Dr. Kamal Polite

DCEM, DOM, AP, CHE

Copyright

This book is intended for educational and informational purposes only. It does not provide medical advice and is not intended to diagnose, treat, cure, or prevent any disease. For full details regarding scope and limitations, please refer to the Medical Disclaimer.

Published by
OHO Publishing
Winter Park, FL, USA

ISBN: 979-8-9947506-1-2
Printed in the United States of America

OHO
Publishing

MERIDIAN & ORGAN TIMES

The Twelve-Hour Cycles, Outer Ring and Inner Ring

The outer ring shows Meridian Time, the peak flow of Qi through the surface channel pathways. The inner ring shows Organ Time, when the physical organs are most metabolically active. The two sequences are offset by approximately two hours.

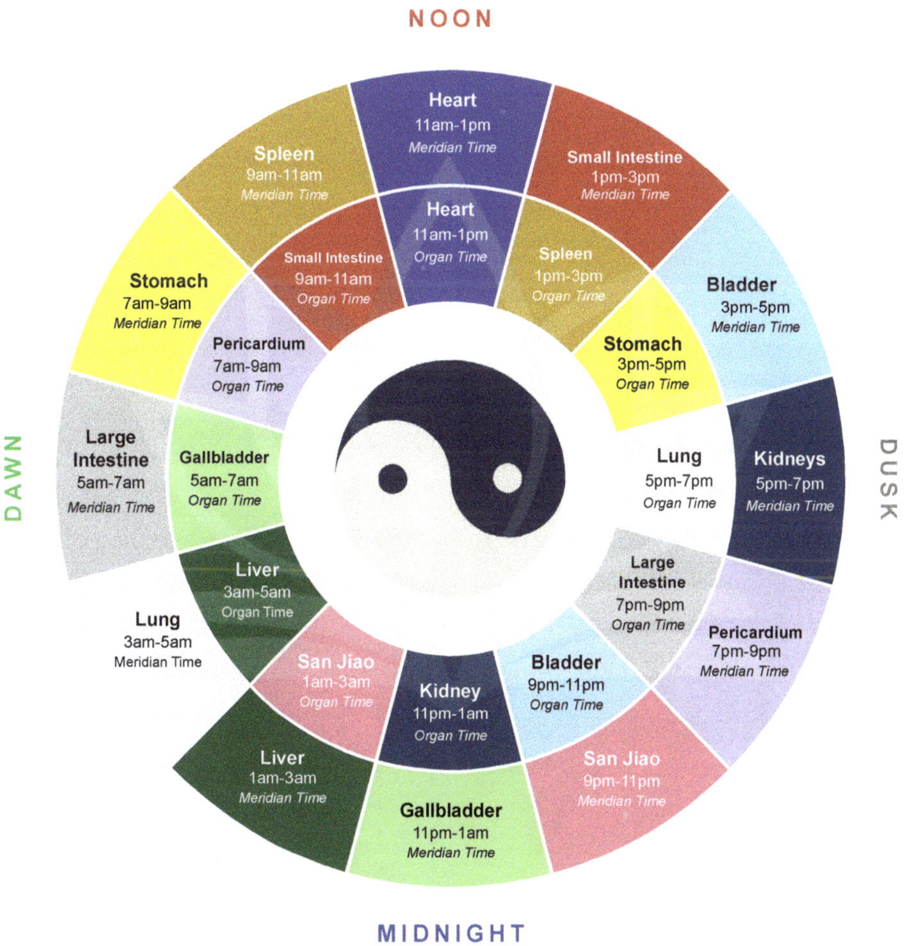

Medical Disclaimer

The material presented here is intended for educational and informational purposes only. It is not intended to diagnose, treat, cure, or prevent any disease. The information reflects integrative perspectives on health, laboratory interpretation, physiology, and timing and is not a substitute for professional medical advice, diagnosis, or treatment.

Always seek the guidance of a qualified healthcare professional with any questions you may have regarding a medical condition, laboratory results, symptoms, or treatment decisions. Never disregard professional medical advice or delay seeking it because of something you have read in this book.

The author does not make claims regarding individual outcomes. Health conditions, responses, and medical needs vary widely based on genetics, environment, lifestyle, and medical history. Any examples discussed are for educational illustration only.

Table of Contents

PREFACE

Author’s Note

These pages were written for patients who have been told their blood tests are “within range,” yet continue to experience unexplained symptoms that do not correspond with the interpretation of current Western medical standards.

Over the course of my clinical career, I have met countless patients who sensed that something in their body was not functioning according to their normal, even when standard laboratory testing failed to provide answers. Their frustration was rooted in not being heard within the current medical system — falling into the gap between lived experience and how laboratory data is commonly interpreted.

My training took place in both Western clinical environments and Chinese Medicine hospital systems, most notably during my time at 山东烟台比尔 Yuhuangding Hospital in Yantai, Shandong, where I trained during the summer of 1996. There, I witnessed how timing, observation, and restraint shaped clinical outcomes as much as anatomy or pharmacology. Blood was not treated as static. Physiology was understood as rhythmic synergy.

This book does not contend with current Western medical standards. On the contrary, it respects their contemporary understanding. As I often joke with my Western-trained colleagues, "Everything you learned in medical training is exactly correct, it's just not always useful." Western laboratory science is precise, indispensable, and lifesaving. What it often lacks is context — particularly temporal context.

One source of that missing context is the framework used throughout this book: Organ Time — the clinical timing system applied in hospital-based Chinese Medicine practice, which describes when the physical organs themselves are most physiologically active. This is not the organ clock you will find if you search online. The version commonly circulated assigns the wrong organ to nearly every time window, because it maps surface meridian pathways rather than actual organ activity. The distinction is not academic. It changes which laboratory values are most meaningful at which hour, which symptoms point to which systems, and what your blood draw — taken almost always in the morning — is and is not capable of capturing. Understanding that distinction is a significant part of what this book offers.

The purpose here is to help patients understand what blood tests can and cannot reveal, how timing influences interpretation, and how classical Chinese Medicine frameworks can add clarity without replacing conventional Western medical standards.

If this book helps you ask better questions, feel more confident in medical conversations, or better understand your own physiology, then it has fulfilled its purpose.

Dr. Kamal

PREFACE

Acknowledgments

Medicine, at its best, is something you absorb more than you are taught. This book is the result of thirty years of that kind of learning — from teachers who demonstrated rather than declared, from patients who asked better questions than I had answers for, and from clinical environments that made it clear, early, that the body always knows more than the chart.

I would like to acknowledge the physicians, staff, and institutional culture of Florida College of Integrated Medicine, where I completed a three-calendar-year, four-academic-year program and was part of the first cohort to travel to China as part of a formal clinical exchange. That visit led to Yuhuangding Hospital entering a sister-institution relationship with FCIM that lasted for several years — a quiet but meaningful bridge between two medical traditions that did not need to be in opposition.

That exchange brought me to 山东烟台比尔 Yuhuangding Hospital in Yantai, Shandong in the summer of 1996, and it radically changed my understanding of the human body. I arrived with a broad foundation in Classical Chinese Medicine and, if I am honest, a somewhat limited exposure to Western clinical practice in a hospital setting. What I was hoping to find was an ancient culture preserved in amber. What I found instead was a fully functioning modern hospital where Classical Chinese Medicine principles were not a separate department — they were woven into daily clinical rounds, into the reading of blood tests and EKGs and imaging, into treatment decisions made in real time with real patients. The physicians there did not explain themselves often. This is not a Western curriculum. Water is only wet when you dive in, and boy were we thrown in the deep end of the pool.

What Yuhuangding gave me was not a philosophy. It was fluency. The Western clinical picture — laboratory values, diagnostic imaging, cardiac monitoring — completed itself for me inside that hospital, not as a separate track from Chinese Medicine but as part of the same unbroken practice. There was no East. There was no West. There was medicine, with every available tool on the table, and a clear pathway toward recovery. That is the standard this book is written to.

I am deeply grateful to the patients who have entrusted me with their care over the last three decades. They are the reason this book exists and the reason it needed to be written plainly. Their persistence in the face of being told "your labs are normal" when their bodies were clearly telling a different story — that persistence was a cry for help. It is intelligence, and that drive for self-advocacy earned my deep respect. They knew something was being missed. They were correct. Their questions shaped this work far more than any theory or principle ever could, and what holds true in practice has always, without exception, come from them first. Patients are the reason physicians exist.

Finally, I acknowledge the Ancient Chinese Medicine traditions that have carried these principles forward across millennia like a precious treasure that never diminishes in value — traditions that emphasize humility, clarity, and patience, and that understand health as something to be recognized and supported, not prescribed to people who were never given a choice.

INTRODUCTION

When Time Became Clinical

子午流注 — Zǐ Wǔ Liú Zhù

My enduring relationship with 子午流注 (Zǐ Wǔ Liú Zhù), Midnight-Noon Ebb-Flow, did not begin in a library. It began on a hospital ward in Yantai, Shandong, in the summer of 1996, where I watched it being used on actual patients by physicians who had never stopped using it — because in that environment, no one had ever suggested they should.

I had completed my training at Florida College of Integrated Medicine — a program with roots stretching back to the John Shen Institute of Chinese Medicine, a lineage that took classical transmission seriously. The program was rigorous, and my foundation in Classical Chinese Medicine was solid. My exposure to Western clinical practice in a hospital setting, however, was limited. That was about to change in ways I did not anticipate.

I was part of the first cohort from FCIM to travel to China as part of a formal clinical exchange. That visit resulted in Yuhuangding Hospital entering a sister-institution relationship with FCIM — a bridge between two traditions that, as

I was about to discover, had never actually been separate in the first place.

Yuhuangding Hospital in Yantai is a regional medical and teaching hospital founded in 1890. By the time I arrived, it had been operating as a fully integrated clinical institution for over a century — not integrated in the way that word is used cautiously in Western healthcare, as though two systems are being introduced to each other across a negotiating table, but integrated in the way that a kitchen is integrated: every tool available, used according to what the situation requires, without ideological preference for the knife over the spoon.

What I encountered there reframed everything I thought I understood about both systems. Blood tests, EKGs, imaging, clinical rounds — the full apparatus of Western diagnostic medicine was in use daily, read and interpreted by physicians who also understood pulse diagnosis, tongue presentation, and the temporal frameworks of Classical Chinese Medicine. These were not two separate departments consulting each other. They were one department, using one language, asking one question: what does this patient need, and when?

That last word — when — is what this book is about.

THE PRESENCE OF 田文 — TIÁN WÉN

This encounter unfolded under the institutional leadership of 田文 (Tián Wén), the hospital president at that time and an integrative physician whose authority expressed itself quietly rather than demonstratively. His presence carried 神

(Shén) — not as mysticism, but as clarity. The kind of clarity that does not need to announce itself.

Even with limited linguistic fluency on my part, understanding arrived. Not through translation, and not through explanation — through demonstration. You watched, and you understood. You waited, and you understood that too. One did not need to be told when to wait; one sensed it. Leadership, I learned there, is recognized rather than declared. It was one of many things that hospital taught me that no curriculum had.

What left the strongest impression was the absence of spectacle. No claims were made. No doctrine was defended. These principles had been applied since the classical era, and the results were simply allowed to speak. That restraint was itself instructive — it demonstrated something I have carried into every clinical encounter since: that what is genuinely effective does not require a sales pitch.

子午流注 — A NOTE ON TIME IN MEDICINE

Within this environment, Zi Wu Liu Zhu was not presented as an abstract clock theory. It was principle realized. Treatment timing influenced outcomes in ways that exceeded anatomical explanation. Channel access, needle sequencing, and therapeutic emphasis shifted according to the hour, and those shifts produced clinically discernible differences. The same diagnosis treated at different times was not the same treatment. That is not a philosophical position. It is an observation that holds up clinically.

From that experience, I later offered my students a phrase: "Let principles be your practice, as your practice reveals the principles." It is easy to read Zi Wu Liu Zhu as theory. It is something else entirely to watch a physician adjust a treatment protocol at 2 PM because the window for that intervention has passed, and to see the patient respond differently as a result. At that point, it stops being theory.

子午流注 — ZǏ WǓ LIÚ ZHÙ: WHAT IT MEANS

子 (Zǐ) — Midnight

午 (Wǔ) — Noon

流 (Liú) — Flow

注 (Zhù) — Infusion or Circulation

Together: the continuous flow of vitality through the body from midnight to noon and back again — a 24-hour cycle in which each organ system has a period of peak physiological activity, and in which the timing of observation, intervention, or blood collection carries clinical meaning.

Zi Wu Liu Zhu is a classical framework in Chinese Medicine that describes how physiological activity moves through the body in a predictable, time-based sequence structured around twelve double-hours (时辰, shí chen), which together span the full day and night. Rather than viewing the body as static, it understands physiology as rhythmic — vital processes rise, peak, and recede according to time, much like the tides. Timing, in this context, is not symbolic. It is functional.

The framework is sometimes simplified as an "organ clock," but that phrase understates its clinical precision. It informs decisions about when to observe, when to intervene, and when to wait. In practice, it functions less as a rulebook and more as a listening framework — one that accounts for temporal patterns that time-independent models of care routinely overlook.

Its principles emerged from the same intellectual lineage that produced the 黄帝内经 Huángdì Nèijīng — the foundational classical text in which medicine was inseparable from astronomy, calendrics, and the observation of cyclical time. Health was understood not as a fixed state but as a dynamic process governed by predictable rhythms. By the Ming dynasty, Zi Wu Liu Zhu was regarded as an advanced discipline, taught only after foundational diagnostic skills had been mastered. Its use required restraint, careful observation, and sensitivity to pattern rather than reliance on standardized protocols.

As modern medicine increasingly emphasized time-neutral models of physiology, this form of temporal reasoning became less prominent in formal Western training. Yet in clinical environments where the tradition remained intact — Yuhuangding among them — Zi Wu Liu Zhu continued to function as a living system. Timing was not theoretical. It was observed, tested, and confirmed through experience, daily, on patients who got better.

ONE FRAMEWORK, TWO VERSIONS — AND WHY IT MATTERS

There is something important to address before you go any further — particularly if you have already searched online for information about Chinese Medicine organ timing, because there is a good chance what you found was incomplete. Not wrong exactly, but pointed at the wrong ring of the clock.

The framework commonly circulated online and in most introductory Chinese Medicine texts is Meridian Time — a sequence describing the peak flow of Qi through the surface channel pathways. It assigns the Gallbladder to 11 PM–1 AM, the Liver to 1–3 AM, the Lung to 3–5 AM, and so on. This is a real framework with real clinical applications, primarily in acupuncture point selection and needle timing.

It is not, however, what this book uses. And it is not what was applied at Yuhuangding.

The clinical framework used throughout this book is Organ Time — the inner ring of the cycle, which describes when the physical organs themselves are most metabolically and physiologically active. These two sequences are offset by approximately two hours, and the clinical consequences of that offset are not minor.

The simplest illustration: according to Meridian Time, 11 PM to 1 AM is Gallbladder time. According to Organ Time, 11 PM to 1 AM is Kidney time. If you wake consistently in that window needing to urinate, Meridian Time points you toward bile secretion and gallbladder function. Organ Time — and Western renal physiology — points you directly at the kidneys, which are genuinely at their peak filtration and hormonal activity in that window. Creatinine and urinalysis results drawn near that time reflect actual kidney activity at its most expressive. The pattern is not philosophical. It is anatomical.

> *What most organ clock resources show you is the surface. This book works from the inside out.*

This distinction is one of the missing halves this book is here to provide. When you understand which organ is actually active at the hour your blood was drawn, the numbers on your report begin to mean something different — more specific, more personal, and more useful than a reference range alone can tell you.

HOW THIS BOOK PROCEEDS

In my Western biomedical training, I was taught to trust the blood before the patient. Too often, subjective complaints were set aside when laboratory values appeared unremarkable. What I came to understand — first at Yuhuangding, and then across three decades of clinical practice — is that what patients were expressing was often already present in the data. The data just needed to be read at the right time, in the right context, with the right framework.

Zi Wu Liu Zhu ceased to be allegorical the moment I watched it work. It became a method of strategic clinical observation, refining the examination process and deepening the ability to correlate findings across patients, physiology, and time. This book proceeds from that lived encounter.

The chapters that follow will move through the most commonly ordered laboratory panels — the CBC, the metabolic panel, lipids, inflammatory markers, hormones — and show how each one reads differently when timing, context, and Organ Time are part of the interpretation. The goal is not to replace your physician's analysis. It is to give you the part of the conversation that most lab reports leave out.

You have been handed a document that describes your body at one specific moment in time. This book is going to help you understand what that moment actually means — and what it cannot tell you on its own.

That is the missing half.

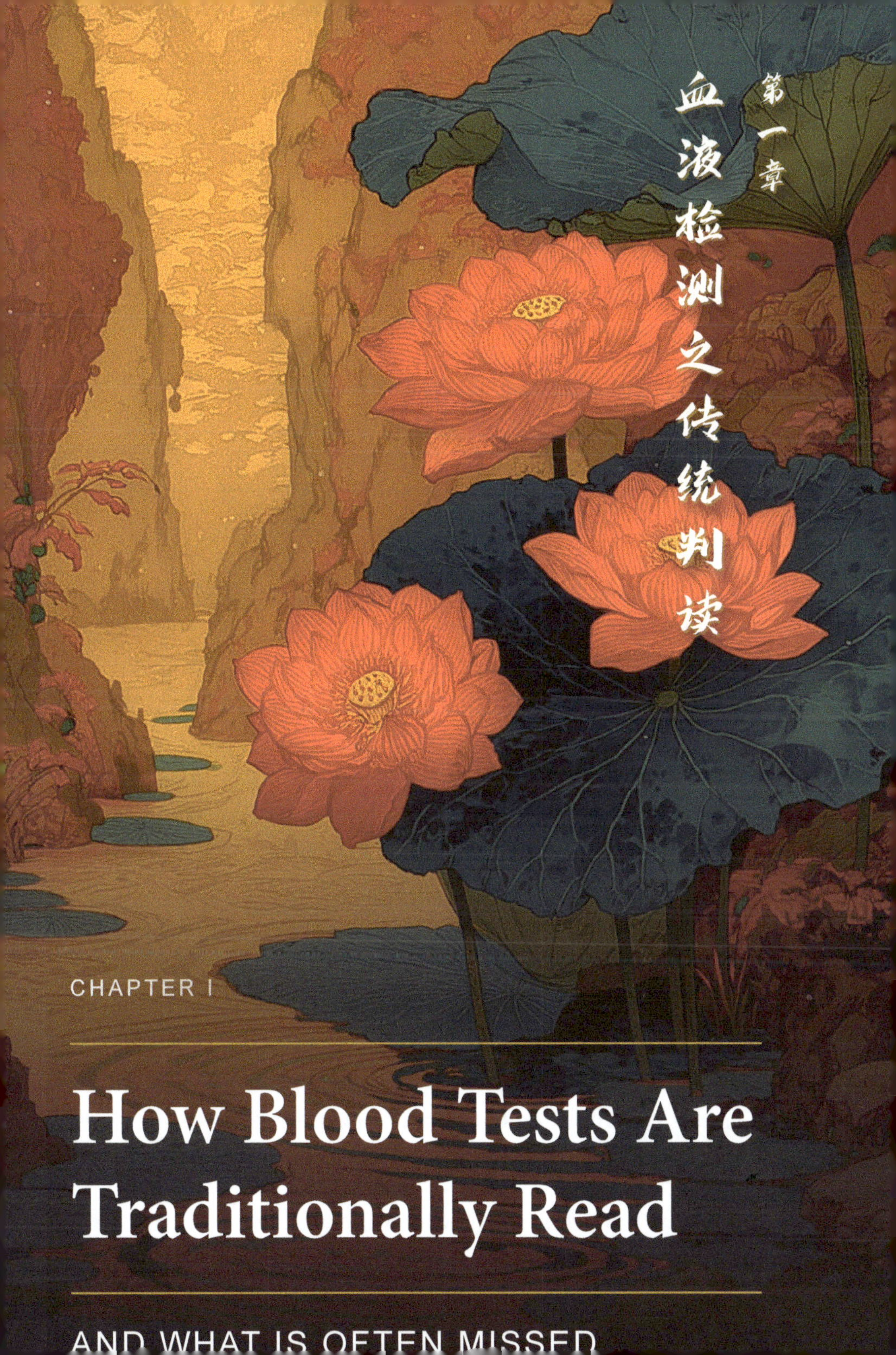

第一章

血液检测之传统判读

CHAPTER I

How Blood Tests Are Traditionally Read

AND WHAT IS OFTEN MISSED

How Blood Tests Are Traditionally Read

AND WHAT IS OFTEN MISSED

Let's start with something most people already sense but haven't been given language for.

You go in for blood work. The results come back. Everything is "within range." Your physician is reassured. You are told there is nothing to worry about. And yet — you still feel exactly the way you felt before you walked in. The fatigue is still there. The brain fog is still there. The sense that something is not quite right is still there. You leave with a clean report and an unanswered question.

That gap — between what the numbers show and what your body is telling you — is not your imagination. It is not anxiety. It is not a failure of modern medicine. It is a gap in interpretation, and it has a specific cause: blood tests are almost always read as though the body exists outside of time.

They do not account for when the blood was drawn. They do not account for what the body was doing at that moment. They do not account for which organ system was at its peak activity, which was at rest, and which was quietly compensating for something that will not show up on a report for another six months. They capture one frame from a continuous film and hand it to you as the whole story.

This chapter is about why that happens, what it misses, and what becomes possible when you read that frame with its full context restored.

> *A blood test is not a portrait of your health.*
> *It is a photograph taken at a specific moment,*
> *under specific conditions, by a camera*
> *pointed in one direction.*

WHAT WESTERN MEDICINE IS DESIGNED TO FIND

Western laboratory medicine is one of the most powerful diagnostic tools ever developed. This is not a criticism of it — it is an acknowledgment of what it was built to do, and what it does extraordinarily well.

It was built to find disease. Specifically, it was built to answer one question with clarity and speed: is there evidence of structural failure, acute danger, or pathological process that requires intervention right now? When the answer is yes, Western laboratory medicine is indispensable. It identifies infection, anemia, organ failure, metabolic crisis, autoimmune activity, and malignancy. It saves lives every day.

That is not a small thing.

The limitation is not in the tool. It is in the question. When the answer to "is there disease present?" is no, the system tends toward reassurance. Reference ranges — the printed intervals beside each value on your report — are derived from population averages. They tell you whether your value falls within the range where most people's values fall. What they do not tell you is whether your body is maintaining that value with ease or with effort. Whether it has been trending quietly in one direction for two years. Whether it looks different at 8 AM than it does at 4 PM. Whether the organ responsible for producing or regulating that value was at its peak or its lowest point when your blood was collected.

Reference ranges describe the boundary of the common. They do not describe the terrain inside it.

WHAT CHINESE MEDICINE IS DESIGNED TO NOTICE

Chinese Medicine approaches the same data from a different starting position. Rather than first asking whether the body is failing, it asks how the body is functioning. Is the system strained? Is it compensating? Is it mis-timed?

These are not vague questions. They have specific clinical answers that produce specific clinical decisions. A value within reference range may still reflect increased effort — the body working harder than it should have to, just to hold a number in place. A hormone produced in adequate quantity but released at the wrong hour may function poorly despite appearing normal on paper. Inflammatory activity may be present and meaningful but entirely unmeasured if it peaks outside the window in which blood was drawn.

This is not philosophy. It is physiology observed across time, applied in hospital settings, and confirmed through clinical outcomes. At Yuhuangding Hospital in Yantai, where I trained in 1996, blood was not treated as a static document. It was understood as a time-sensitive expression of a body in motion. Laboratory values were correlated with the Four Examinations — looking, listening, asking, and touching — and interpreted in the context of when they were collected, what the patient was experiencing, and where those values sat within the body's daily physiological rhythm.

The result was a form of interpretation that neither system could produce alone. Western laboratory precision, read through the lens of temporal physiology. Numbers with their context intact.

> *Western Medicine and Chinese Medicine are not looking at different bodies. They are looking at the same body from different distances — and at different times of day.*

THE MISSING VARIABLE: TIME

Consider what your standard blood draw actually captures. In most clinical settings, blood is collected in the early morning, fasting, before the day's demands have begun.

This standardization is practical and useful — it improves comparability between draws and reduces some variables. But it introduces a different variable that almost no one accounts for: every value on your report reflects what your body was doing at that specific hour, in that specific physiological state, during that specific phase of a 24-hour cycle that never stops moving.

Cortisol — the body's primary timing and stress-response hormone — can vary by a factor of five or six between its morning peak and its midnight low. A cortisol value drawn at 8 AM and one drawn at 8 PM in the same person, on the same day, will look like they belong to two different patients. Testosterone follows a similar pattern, declining 25 to 50 percent between early morning and late afternoon. Thyroid-stimulating hormone peaks around midnight and reaches its lowest point in the mid-afternoon. Inflammatory markers, iron levels, and immune activity all shift meaningfully across the day.

None of this variation is recorded on your lab report. None of it is typically considered in interpretation. The number is the number, regardless of when it was taken.

This is where Organ Time — the clinical framework at the heart of this book — becomes practically relevant. Not as an ancient curiosity, but as a diagnostic lens that accounts for what the body was doing at the moment your blood was drawn, and what that context means for the value you are now being asked to interpret.

A Simple Example

You wake consistently between 11 PM and 1 AM needing to urinate. Your morning creatinine and kidney function markers come back normal. Most online organ clock resources will tell you that 11 PM–1 AM is Gallbladder time — and point you toward bile secretion and liver detoxification.

Organ Time — the clinical inner-ring sequence used in hospital-based Chinese Medicine practice and throughout this book — assigns 11 PM to 1 AM to the Kidneys. Western renal physiology agrees: the kidneys are at peak filtration and hormonal activity in this window. Your symptom is not incidental. It is the kidney system expressing itself at its most active hour. The fact that your morning creatinine looks normal does not mean the kidneys are unstressed — it means the blood was drawn when the kidneys were at rest, not when they were at work.

That is the difference timing makes.

HOW TO READ THIS BOOK

The chapters that follow move through the most commonly ordered laboratory panels: the Complete Blood Count, the Metabolic Panel, Lipids, Inflammatory Markers, and Hormones. Each chapter presents what Western Medicine observes in that panel, what Classical Chinese Medicine adds to that observation, and — crucially — how the timing of the draw shapes what the numbers mean.

This is not a book that will tell you what is wrong with you. It is a book that will help you understand what your blood work is actually saying, what it is not equipped to say, and what questions are worth asking when the report comes back and the gap between the numbers and your experience refuses to close.

You already sensed something was missing. You were right. Let's look at what it is.

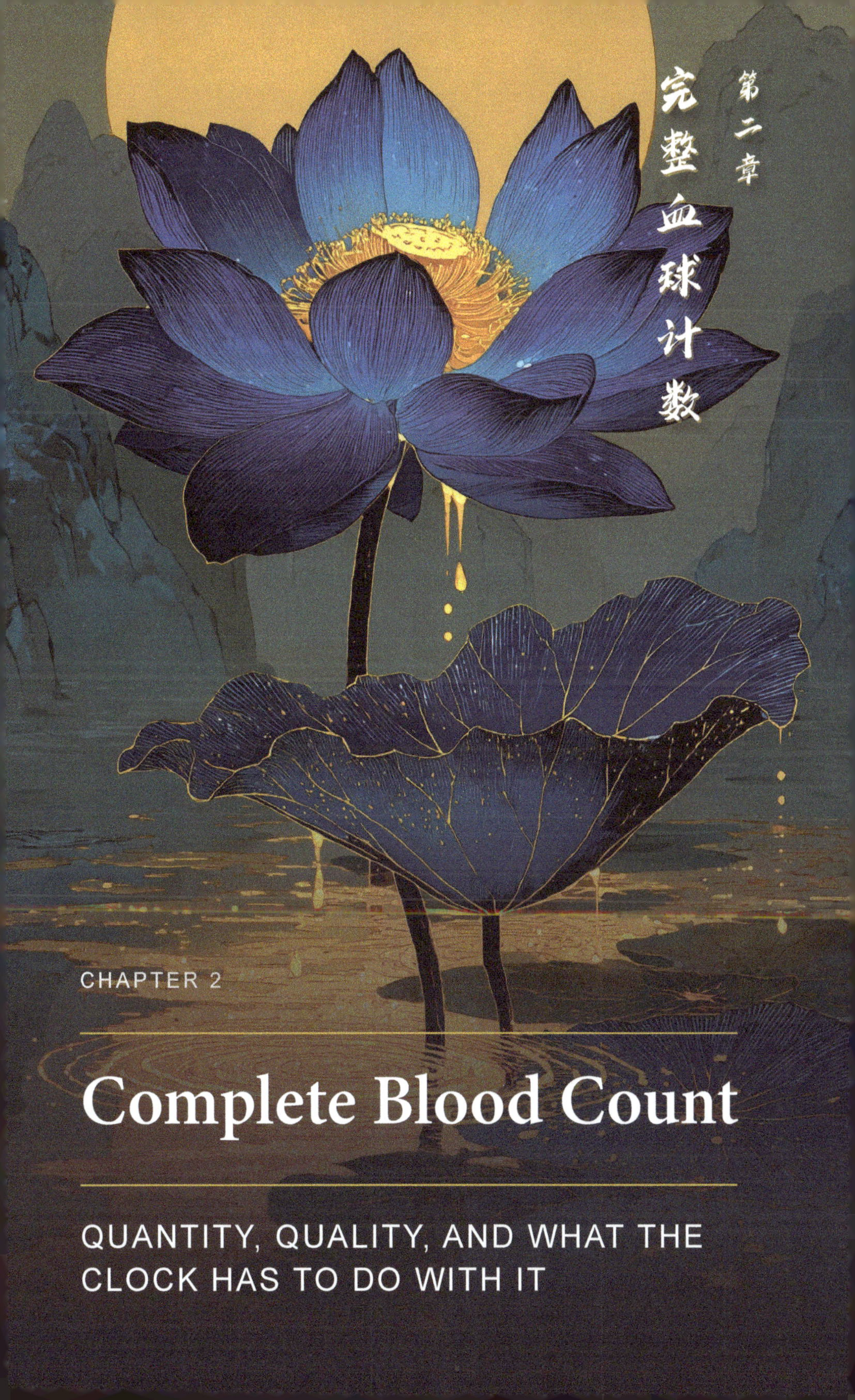

第二章
完整血球计数

CHAPTER 2

Complete Blood Count

QUANTITY, QUALITY, AND WHAT THE CLOCK HAS TO DO WITH IT

Complete Blood Count

QUANTITY, QUALITY, AND WHAT THE CLOCK HAS TO DO WITH IT

The Complete Blood Count — the CBC — is probably the test you've had ordered more times than any other. It is routine in the way that a morning check-in is routine: quick, standardized, and easy to overlook precisely because it happens so often. But routine does not mean simple, and familiar does not mean fully understood.

The CBC evaluates three primary populations of cells in your blood: red blood cells, which carry oxygen to every tissue in the body; white blood cells, which coordinate immune response and defense; and platelets, which govern clotting and tissue repair. Together they offer a snapshot of how well the body is delivering what it needs, defending what it has, and recovering from what it encounters.

That word — snapshot — is doing a lot of work. And as we established in Chapter 1, the hour that snapshot was taken matters more than most reports acknowledge. The CBC is no exception. Before we get into what each value means, it is worth understanding what each system is designed to see when it looks at these numbers — because Western Medicine and Chinese Medicine are not asking the same question when they read the same report.

WHAT WESTERN MEDICINE READS IN THE CBC

From a Western perspective, the CBC is primarily a screening tool — precise, reproducible, and calibrated to identify when something has crossed into clinical danger. The red blood cell indices are used to classify anemia by type, which in turn points toward cause and treatment. The white blood cell count detects infection, immune suppression, or hematologic disease. Platelets flag clotting risk in either direction.

The anemia classifications are worth understanding in some detail, because they illustrate both the precision of Western laboratory medicine and its timing limitation.

Microcytic Anemia

Characterized by red blood cells that are smaller than normal. The most common cause is iron deficiency, though it also appears in chronic blood loss, thalassemia, and long-standing inflammatory states. Symptoms — fatigue, cold sensitivity, shortness of breath, weakness — are often present for months or years before hemoglobin levels fall below diagnostic thresholds. The body compensates quietly for a long time before the numbers catch up. By the time the CBC flags it, the patient has usually already been living with it.

Normocytic Anemia

Red blood cells are normal in size but reduced in overall oxygen-carrying capacity. This pattern is commonly associated with chronic disease, kidney dysfunction, acute blood loss, or bone marrow suppression. Because cell size appears normal, this form of anemia is frequently underappreciated despite producing significant symptoms. It does not announce itself with an obvious morphological flag. It simply reduces the body's capacity, quietly, until the patient is running at 70 percent with no clear explanation.

Macrocytic Anemia

Red blood cells are larger than normal, often linked to vitamin B12 or folate deficiency, alcohol use, liver disease, or medication effects. Neurological symptoms — numbness, cognitive changes, mood disturbance — can precede significant changes in hemoglobin values, sometimes by years. The CBC catches this category well once the morphological change is established. The challenge, again, is that the change establishes itself slowly while the patient experiences the consequences in advance of the flag.

> *Western classification of anemia is precise and necessary. Its limitation is not accuracy — it is timing. The CBC identifies what has already happened. Chinese Medicine looks for what is still becoming.*

White blood cells are evaluated by total count and, when ordered, by differential — the relative proportions of neutrophils, lymphocytes, monocytes, eosinophils, and basophils. Absolute counts detect active infection or immune suppression. Elevated counts point toward acute response; suppressed counts may indicate bone marrow compromise, viral illness, or the body's reserves running thin. Platelets flag clotting risk: too low suggests bleeding tendency or bone marrow strain; too high may reflect inflammatory activity or reactive production following stress or surgery.

This is a powerful and clinically essential framework. Where it becomes less informative is in the borderline zone — values that are within range but trending, values that are low-normal when the patient's symptoms suggest they should be higher, values that look stable on paper while the patient feels anything but.

WHAT CHINESE MEDICINE READS IN THE CBC

Chinese Medicine does not classify anemia by cell size. It evaluates Blood (血, Xuè) as a living substance that must be sufficient in quantity, sound in quality, and able to move freely through the body. These are three different problems with three different presentations — and all three can exist while the CBC remains technically within reference range.

Blood Deficiency

Not simply low hemoglobin — Blood Deficiency describes a state in which the body's nourishing capacity is insufficient relative to its demands. Fatigue that worsens with mental effort, dizziness upon standing, dry skin, poor concentration, palpitations at rest, and a quality of anxiety that feels more like emptiness than agitation — these are Blood Deficiency presentations. They can appear when hemoglobin is 13.5 g/dL just as readily as when it is 10. The number alone does not tell you whether the blood is nourishing adequately. The patient's experience does.

Blood Stagnation

Blood is present but not moving efficiently. Fixed pain, headaches that return to the same location, clotting tendencies, a complexion that looks dull rather than pale — these reflect stagnation rather than deficiency. Platelet counts may appear normal. The issue is not quantity but circulation. In Chinese Medicine, the Liver governs the smooth movement of Blood; when Liver function is strained — by chronic stress, emotional suppression, or sustained physical demand — Blood begins to pool rather than flow.

Heat in the Blood

Inflammatory, restless, or agitated presentations — skin eruptions, excessive menstrual bleeding, a quality of heat that moves rather than stays fixed — despite white blood cell counts that appear normal. Heat in the Blood is not infection as Western Medicine defines it. It is a state of excitation in the circulatory system that can drive symptoms without crossing the numerical threshold that would flag a white blood cell differential.

On Defensive Qi — Wèi Qì (卫气)

White blood cells in Chinese Medicine are understood through the lens of Wei Qi (卫气,Wèi Qì) — Defensive Qi — the body's surface protection and first-line immune response. Chronically elevated white blood cell count may reflect active defense; chronically suppressed white blood cell count may reflect depletion of that defensive capacity rather than simple immune suppression. The distinction matters clinically because the interventions are different. You do not treat depletion the same way you treat excess. A white blood cell count of 4.1 $x10^9/L$ in a patient who gets every cold that passes through the office is telling a different story than a white blood cell count of 4.1 in someone who is robustly well. Same number. Different body. Different meaning.

WHEN THE CBC WAS DRAWN — AND WHY IT CHANGES THE PICTURE

The CBC is collected in the early morning in most clinical settings. For red blood cell indices — hemoglobin, hematocrit, Mean Corpuscular Volume — this timing is relatively stable; these values do not fluctuate dramatically across the day. But two components of the CBC are meaningfully time-sensitive, and both are routinely under-discussed.

Iron — which drives red blood cell production and is frequently evaluated alongside the CBC — follows one of the most pronounced diurnal rhythms of any commonly tested value. Serum iron is typically 30 to 50 percent higher in the morning than in the late afternoon. A patient whose iron is drawn at 8 AM may appear borderline adequate. The same patient drawn at 4 PM may appear deficient. If the original diagnosis was made from a morning draw and the follow-up was done in the afternoon, the apparent decline may reflect the clock more than the patient's actual iron status.

White blood cells also vary across the day, with immune activity influenced by the body's circadian rhythm and, in Organ Time, by the specific organ window active at the time of collection. The Small Intestine governs sorting and assimilation during the 9 AM to 11 AM window — the window in which many CBCs are collected after a patient's early morning draw has been processed. Immune reactivity in this window reflects a different phase of the body's defense cycle than one collected during the Liver window at 3 to 5 AM, when detoxification and immune recalibration are most active.

This does not mean every CBC needs to be drawn twice. It means that when CBC values are borderline, when symptoms and numbers don't agree, or when trends across multiple draws seem inconsistent, the time of collection is a variable worth examining before assuming the numbers are the whole story.

The CBC is not a verdict. It is a time-stamped observation of a body that was doing something specific at the moment the needle went in.

READING THE CBC AS A COMPLETE PICTURE

CBCs rarely tell the complete story on their own. The most informative readings have always come from correlating laboratory values with what the patient is actually experiencing — the quality of their fatigue, the timing of their symptoms, the way they look and carry themselves when they walk in. A pale complexion, a thin pulse, and a hemoglobin of 12.1 g/dL in a woman who reports waking exhausted every morning tells a different story than a hemoglobin of 12.1 in someone who feels well. The number is the starting point, not the conclusion. That is as true today in clinical practice as it was in the hospital wards of Yantai in 1996.

That is the integrated reading this book is building toward. Not a replacement for Western laboratory precision, but an expansion of it — one that accounts for quality alongside quantity, movement alongside presence, and time alongside value.

The CBC tells you what is in your blood. What it does not tell you — on its own — is whether what is there is doing its job, whether it is moving freely, and whether the hour it was measured captured the body at work or at rest. Those questions belong in the interpretation. They are what the next chapters will continue to develop.

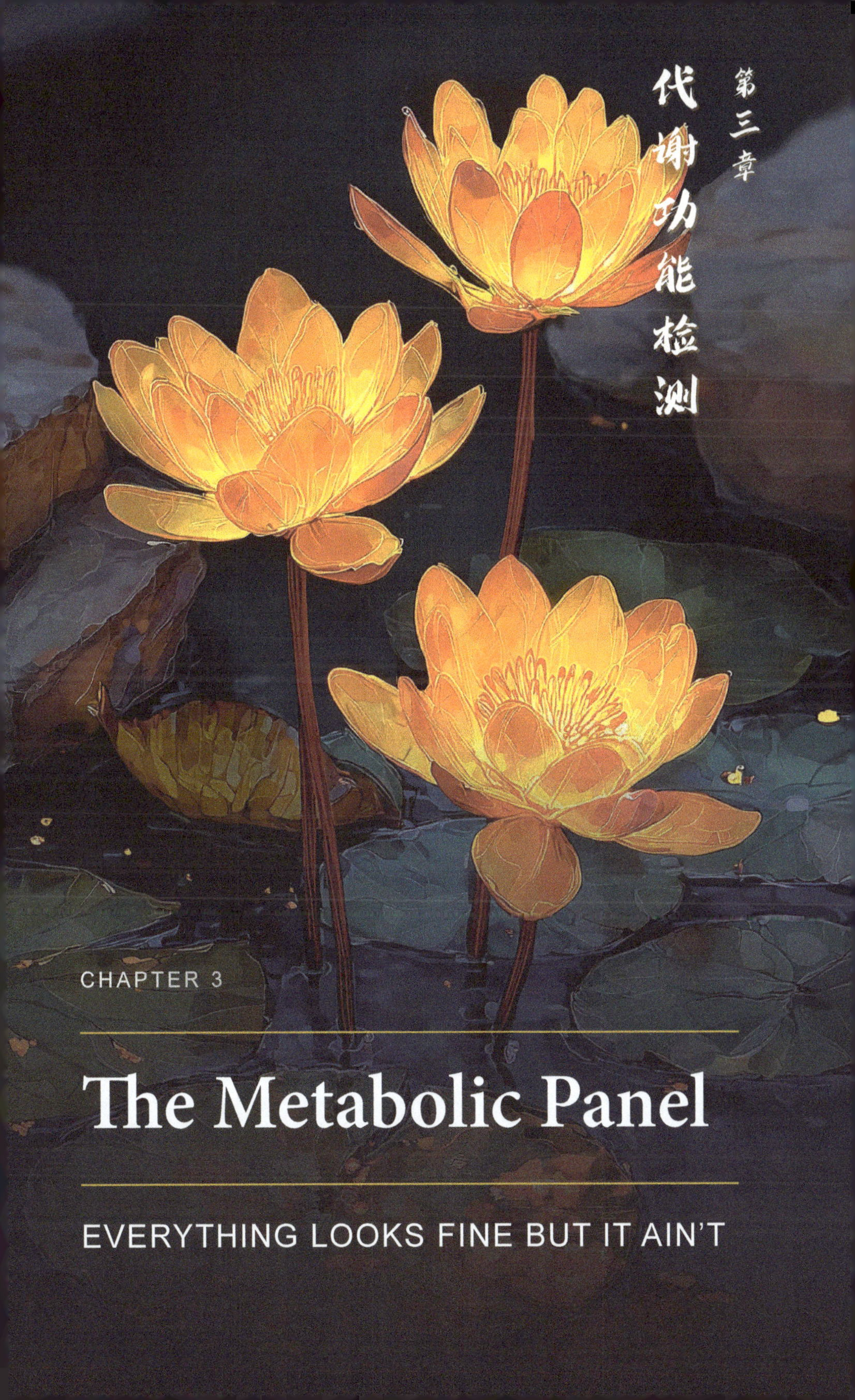

第三章

代谢功能检测

CHAPTER 3

The Metabolic Panel

EVERYTHING LOOKS FINE BUT IT AIN'T

The Metabolic Panel

EVERYTHING LOOKS FINE BUT IT AIN'T

The metabolic panel is the test that most reliably produces the phrase "everything looks fine." It covers the body's most fundamental regulatory functions — fluid balance, mineral levels, energy production, kidney filtration, liver processing — and when those values sit within their reference ranges, the clinical conversation tends to close quickly.

What that conversation often misses is the question underneath the numbers: how much is the body working to keep them there?

A metabolic panel can appear entirely normal while the body is quietly compensating — pulling from reserves, rerouting resources, sustaining balance through effort rather than ease. The panel reflects the outcome of that effort. It does not reflect the effort itself. Learning to read both is what this chapter is about.

> *Normal on a metabolic panel means the body is maintaining regulation. It does not tell you what that maintenance is costing.*

WHAT WESTERN MEDICINE IS LOOKING FOR

The metabolic panel — whether ordered as a Basic Metabolic Panel (BMP) or Comprehensive Metabolic Panel (CMP) — is calibrated to answer one focused question: is there evidence of organ failure or acute physiological distress? When the answer is yes, it answers it well. Severely disrupted electrolytes, markedly elevated creatinine, critically abnormal glucose — these findings direct rapid, appropriate intervention. In that context, the metabolic panel is an essential clinical tool.

Its limitation, as with the CBC, is not accuracy. It is orientation. It is built to find breakdown, not the strain that precedes it.

Electrolytes: Sodium, Potassium, Chloride, Bicarbonate

Electrolytes regulate nerve conduction, muscle contraction, fluid distribution, and acid-base balance. When they move significantly outside reference ranges, the consequences are serious — cardiac arrhythmia, muscle paralysis, respiratory compromise. Western Medicine monitors them precisely for this reason. What the reference range does not capture is the functional significance of values that sit at the edges of normal — the sodium that is technically adequate but reflects chronic dehydration, the potassium that is within range but trending downward in a patient who has been under sustained stress for six months.

Glucose

Fasting glucose screens for diabetes and hypoglycemia. It is a meaningful baseline. What it does not capture is how the body manages energy across the rest of the day — after meals, under stress, in the afternoon when cortisol has declined and insulin sensitivity has shifted. A fasting glucose of 94 mg/dL in the morning can coexist with significant afternoon instability that the patient experiences as crashes, cravings, irritability, and cognitive fog. The morning draw was clean. The afternoon story was never told.

Kidney Markers: Creatinine and Blood Urea Nitrogen

Blood urea nitrogen and creatinine evaluate how efficiently the kidneys are filtering waste. Elevated values indicate reduced filtration capacity; significantly elevated values indicate kidney disease or failure. Within reference range, these markers are generally reassuring — and appropriately so. The nuance comes in the trends. A creatinine that has moved from 0.8 to 1.1 mg/dL over three years, while remaining within range the entire time, is a trend worth noting. The kidney is not failing. But it is working harder than it was. That trajectory matters.

Liver Enzymes: ALT and AST

Alanine aminotransferase (ALT) and aspartate aminotransferase (AST) are markers of liver cell stress. Significant elevations prompt evaluation for hepatitis, medication toxicity, alcohol-related damage, or fatty liver disease. The clinical gap opens in the high-normal range, where values are technically acceptable but persistently elevated. Patients with consistently high-normal ALT have often presented with exactly the constellation of symptoms the liver is responsible for managing: irritability, headaches, bloating, food sensitivities, difficulty processing fats, and an increasing sensitivity to medications at doses that previously caused no issue. The enzymes have not crossed the line. The liver has quietly been running hot for a while.

WHAT CHINESE MEDICINE ADDS TO THIS PICTURE

Chinese Medicine reads the metabolic panel not as a report on organ status, but as a map of functional relationships. The question is not whether an organ has failed — it is whether the system is moving, transforming, and distributing efficiently, and at what cost.

Electrolytes and the Fluid Distribution System

In Chinese Medicine, fluid metabolism is governed primarily by the Lung, Spleen, and Kidney systems working in coordination. The Lung distributes fluids downward and outward; the Spleen transforms and transports them; the Kidney governs their final regulation and storage. When any one of these systems is under strain, fluid distribution becomes inefficient — not absent, but effortful. A sodium value at the low end of normal may reflect chronic Spleen Qi deficiency, where the body's capacity to hold and distribute fluids is weakened. A borderline potassium may reflect the same, or may indicate Yin deficiency — insufficient moisture and containment at the cellular level. These are not diagnoses from a single number. They are questions the number raises when the patient's experience is in the room alongside it.

Glucose, the Liver, and the Energy Regulation Story

This is one of the most clinically instructive relationships in the metabolic panel, and one of the most underappreciated. In Chinese Medicine, the Liver stores Blood (血, Xuè), and Blood is understood as the mother of Qi (气, Qì) — the body's functional energy. The Liver's ability to store and release Blood smoothly is directly related to glycogen storage and glucose availability. When Liver Qi is constrained — by chronic stress, emotional suppression, or sustained physical demand — that smooth release becomes erratic. The body struggles to regulate energy not because glucose is absent, but because the distribution is disrupted.

This is why patients with normal fasting glucose can experience significant energy instability across the day. The morning draw captured the storage state. It did not capture what happens when the Liver is asked to release that energy smoothly under the demands of a full day — and cannot.

Creatinine, Jing, and the Long-Term Reserve Question

Creatinine within range does not always indicate sufficient

Jing (精, Jīng) — the deep constitutional reserve the Kidneys govern in Chinese Medicine. Jing is the body's long-term endowment: the capacity for sustained effort, recovery after illness or stress, and graceful aging. It depletes slowly, over years, and laboratory markers often lag behind its decline.

In clinical practice, patients whose creatinine is trending upward within the normal range — even subtly — while simultaneously reporting declining endurance, slower recovery from exertion, persistent low back soreness, or cold sensitivity below the waist, are describing a Kidney system under increasing load. The number has not crossed any threshold. The body is already telling the story. Sitting across from patients who feel this way while holding normal lab reports has made that pattern unmistakable.

Liver Enzymes and the Cost of Constraint

Where Western Medicine reads ALT and AST primarily as injury markers, Chinese Medicine reads them as flow markers. The Liver governs the smooth coursing of Qi throughout the body — its ability to keep things moving, processing, and clearing. When that function is constrained — by emotional load, by hormonal burden, by the cumulative weight of things unprocessed — the enzymes reflect the effort of containment rather than the damage of failure.

Mild, persistent, high-normal liver enzyme elevations in the absence of obvious structural cause are one of the patterns I watch most carefully in practice. Not because they indicate disease, but because they indicate a system that is working at capacity and has limited reserve for additional demand. The patient who comes in with an alanine aminotransferase (ALT) of 48 U/L, no drinking history, no medications, and a stressful job they've had for four years — that liver is not diseased. But it is telling you something about the cost of how that person is living.

ORGAN TIME AND THE METABOLIC PANEL

The metabolic panel is almost always drawn fasting, in the early morning. This is clinically appropriate for standardization — and it captures the body in its overnight storage and baseline regulation state. What it does not capture is the metabolic story that unfolds across the rest of the day.

Using Organ Time, the morning draw window falls across the Gallbladder (5–7 AM) and Pericardium (7–9 AM) periods — the body transitioning from overnight detoxification into morning cardiovascular mobilization. Glucose at this hour reflects overnight hepatic regulation. Electrolytes reflect the overnight fluid balance state. Kidney markers reflect the tail end of the Kidney's peak activity window, which runs from 11 PM to 1 AM.

This has specific clinical implications. A patient whose most significant symptoms are afternoon energy crashes, evening electrolyte depletion manifesting as muscle cramps, or early morning fatigue consistent with the body struggling to transition out of the overnight Kidney window — that patient's morning metabolic panel may appear entirely reassuring, because the draw was taken when those systems were at rest rather than under the load that produces the symptoms.

The Spleen Window and Afternoon Glucose

The Spleen governs transformation and transportation of acquired essence — the conversion of food and nutrients into usable Qi and Blood. Its peak Organ Time window is 1 to 3 PM, the same period in which many patients experience their most significant energy instability: post-lunch crashes, foggy thinking, sugar cravings, and the inability to sustain concentration.

A fasting glucose drawn at 7 AM does not measure Spleen time. It measures baseline hepatic glucose regulation. The afternoon glucose story — the one the patient is living — requires either a post-prandial draw, continuous glucose monitoring, or at minimum, an HbA1c that reflects the average across a longer period. When afternoon symptoms are present and morning glucose is normal, the Spleen window is the clinical question that has not been answered.

INJURY VERSUS EFFORT — READING BOTH

The title of this chapter is not accidental. Injury and effort are two different states, and they require two different responses. Western Medicine is excellent at identifying injury — the point at which a system has been sufficiently damaged or overwhelmed to produce measurable pathological change. That is where it intervenes, and those interventions are often lifesaving.

Effort is the earlier state. It is the body maintaining its numbers through increasing work, drawing down reserves, compensating quietly before anything crosses a clinical threshold. Chinese Medicine is calibrated to recognize effort. Clinically the patients who arrive in the most distress are rarely the ones whose labs are dramatically abnormal. They are the ones whose labs have looked normal for years while their bodies worked harder and harder to keep them that way.

The metabolic panel, read with both lenses and with the timing of the draw in mind, is a considerably more informative document than "everything looks fine" suggests. It describes the state of the body's most fundamental regulatory systems at one specific moment in its daily cycle. Understanding what that moment represents — and what it cannot show — is the beginning of a more complete clinical picture.

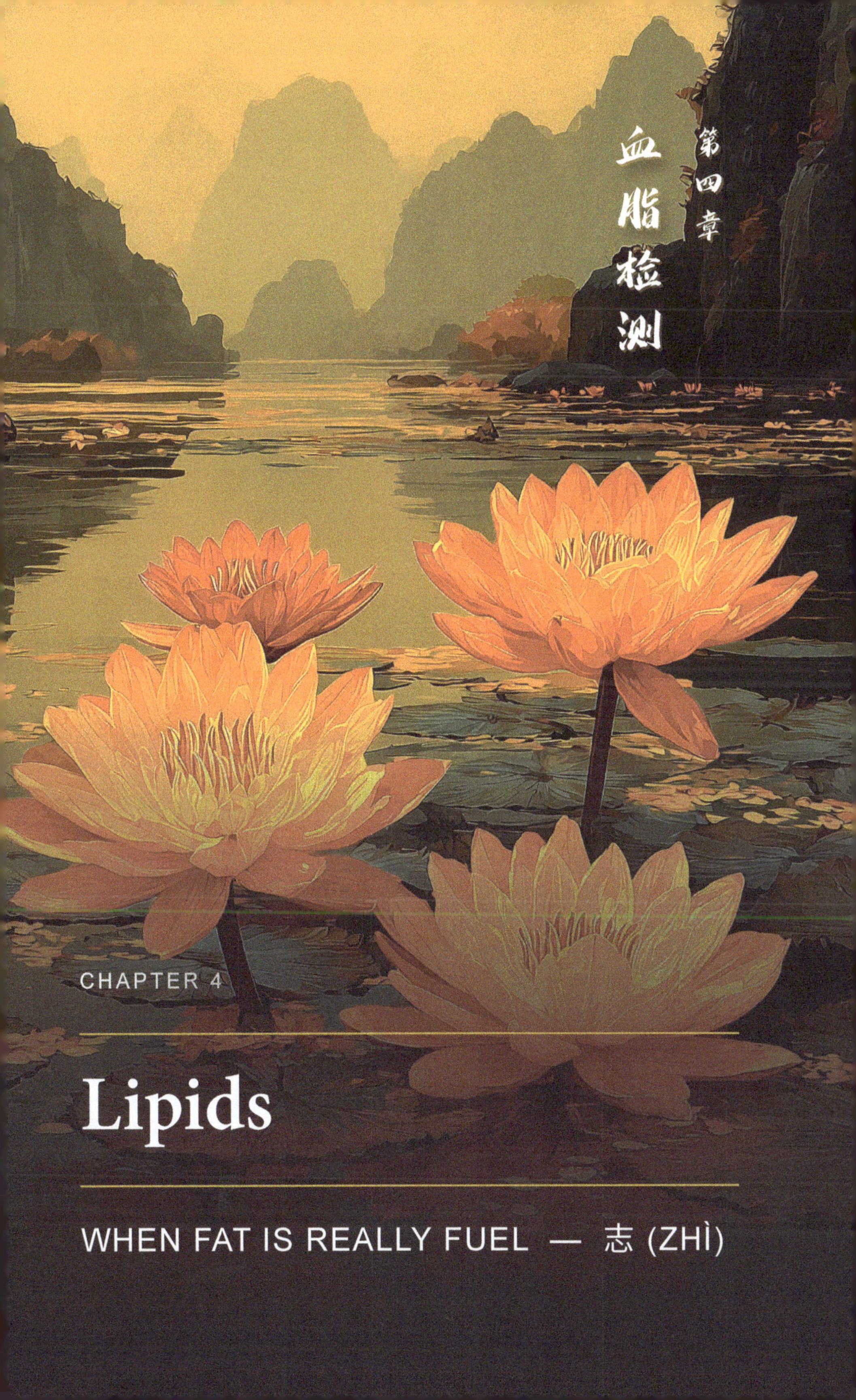

第四章 血脂检测

CHAPTER 4

Lipids

WHEN FAT IS REALLY FUEL — 志 (ZHÌ)

Lipids

WHEN FAT IS REALLY FUEL — 志 (ZHÌ)

Few laboratory results produce more anxiety per number than the lipid panel. Patients come in having already Googled their cholesterol, already convinced that something in the report is trying to kill them, and ready to negotiate their way out of a statin prescription before anyone has said a word. The conversation around lipids has become so compressed — good cholesterol, bad cholesterol, your number is too high — that the actual physiology rarely gets a hearing.

Let's give it one.

Lipids are not toxins. They are materials — essential, purposeful, and produced by a body that knows exactly what it is doing. The body relies on fats to build hormones, insulate nerves, maintain cell membranes, repair damaged tissue, store energy for future demand, and support the structural integrity of every organ in the body. Without lipids, normal physiology cannot be sustained. The question a lipid panel is actually answering is not "is there too much of a dangerous substance?" It is "how is the body managing its most fundamental building material, and does that strategy match the demands being placed on it?"

That is a considerably more interesting question. And it produces considerably more useful answers.

> *Cholesterol is not the villain of this story. Fear of cholesterol, however, has caused a great deal of unnecessary harm — to patients who restricted it when their bodies needed it, and to conversations that ended before they could be useful.*

WHAT THE LIPID PANEL MEASURES

A standard lipid panel includes four values: total cholesterol, low-density lipoprotein (LDL), high-density lipoprotein (HDL), and triglycerides. In Western Medicine, these are used primarily to estimate cardiovascular risk — the likelihood of heart disease or stroke based on population-level correlations between lipid patterns and cardiovascular events. Large epidemiological studies have established these correlations, and they are clinically meaningful at the population level.

The limitation, as with all population-derived reference ranges, is that they are applied uniformly to individuals whose physiological strategies may differ significantly. The body that needs more lipid reserve is not the same body as the one that needs less. Treating them as though they are produces interpretation errors that thirty years of clinical practice have made very familiar.

Total Cholesterol

A broad summary marker. Elevated levels may reflect increased production, impaired clearance, or increased demand for hormone synthesis and tissue repair – the body building more because more is being used or lost. Low total cholesterol, which receives far less attention than it deserves, may reflect malabsorption, chronic illness, nutritional depletion, or a body that has exhausted its manufacturing capacity. Neither direction is inherently problematic without context. Both directions are worth understanding.

Low-Density Lipoprotein (LDL) – The Transport Particle

LDL is not cholesterol. It is a transport particle – a carrier that moves cholesterol from the liver to the tissues that require it for repair, hormone production, and cellular maintenance. It has been labeled "bad cholesterol" in popular culture with such consistency that most patients are genuinely surprised to learn this distinction.

Think of LDL as a bandage. When blood vessels experience ongoing wear, inflammation, or minor damage, the body sends more LDL to deliver the repair materials those tissues need. The bandage is not the problem. The wound is the problem. Elevated LDL in the context of chronic inflammation, hormonal demand, or sustained physical stress is the body doing its job – routing materials to where they are needed. Reading that number without asking why it is elevated is like treating the bandage instead of the injury.

High-Density Lipoprotein (HDL) — The Cleanup Crew

HDL facilitates the return of cholesterol from peripheral tissues back to the liver for reuse or elimination. If LDL is the bandage going out, HDL is the cleanup crew coming back. When repair is efficient, materials are recycled, excess is cleared, and the system maintains itself. Higher HDL levels generally reflect this efficient recovery process. Lower HDL levels may reflect chronic inflammation, metabolic exhaustion, or reduced recovery capacity — a body so occupied with managing ongoing demand that it has little bandwidth left for the cleanup.

Triglycerides — The Stored Fuel

Triglycerides represent energy in storage. When the body takes in more fuel than it can immediately use, it packages the surplus as triglycerides and holds it for later demand. This is not malfunction — it is foresight. The problem arises when the surplus becomes chronic: elevated triglycerides are commonly associated with insulin resistance, disrupted sleep, metabolic stress, and sustained overload. The body is not misbehaving. It is carrying more than it can efficiently use, and that excess accumulates over time.

THE CONSTITUTION QUESTION — A BLOOD TEST FOR A LION IS NOT A BLOOD TEST FOR A HIPPOPOTAMUS

One of the most practically useful concepts in Chinese Medicine is constitutional variation — the understanding that different bodies are built for different physiological strategies, and that what is optimal for one may be inappropriate for another. Nowhere is this more relevant than in lipid interpretation.

Consider two very different animals. A lion is built for speed, intensity, and rapid output. Its physiology favors quick mobilization of energy, efficient circulation, and fast recovery after bursts of activity. Lipid availability needs to be high and responsive. Turnover is rapid. The strategy is readiness.

A hippopotamus is built for endurance, mass, and sustained presence. Its physiology favors conservation, insulation, and long-term reserve. Movement is slower, but stability is paramount. Higher baseline lipid reserves are not a sign of pathology in this body — they are the appropriate strategy for the journey it is built to take.

Neither constitution is healthier by default. They are different designs for different demands. Applied to human physiology: some bodies are built for frequent output and rapid recovery. Others are built for endurance, protection, and long-term resilience. A lipid panel interpreted without any acknowledgment of constitutional type is applying a single standard to a population of individuals whose physiological strategies vary considerably. This is one of the reasons lipid management produces such inconsistent outcomes when applied uniformly.

LIPIDS IN CHINESE MEDICINE — AVAILABILITY, RESERVE, AND 志 (ZHÌ)

In Chinese Medicine, lipid metabolism is understood through the relationship between two organ systems whose functions are distinct but complementary.

The Liver governs availability. It produces, circulates, and distributes lipid material in response to immediate demand — storing Blood so it can be released, keeping fuel accessible so the body can move, respond, and adapt. When the Liver is functioning well, lipids are produced appropriately, distributed efficiently, and cleared when no longer needed. When Liver Qi is constrained — by chronic stress, emotional load, or hormonal burden — that smooth distribution is disrupted. Production may increase as the body tries to compensate for inefficient delivery. Clearance may slow. The lipid panel reflects the congestion.

The Kidney governs reserve. It answers the longer question: how much does this body need to hold in storage for the journey ahead? This is the constitutional layer — the body's assessment of its own endurance requirements, shaped by genetics, history, environment, and the accumulated weight of how life has been lived. A body that has experienced chronic scarcity, sustained stress, or prolonged illness may hold higher lipid reserves not because something has gone wrong, but because its Kidney system has assessed the terrain as uncertain and prepared accordingly.

This is the meaning of 志 (Zhì) — the virtue associated with

the Kidney system. Often translated as will or resolve, Zhì in its clinical expression is the quiet capacity to hold the long view: to conserve without panic, to sustain without depletion, to carry what the journey requires without being overwhelmed by it. When lipid values are read through this lens, elevated reserves are not automatically a warning. They are a question worth asking: what is this body preparing for, and does the preparation match the actual demand?

The Liver and Kidney in Lipid Terms

The Liver packs what is needed for today — producing and distributing lipid material in response to immediate demand, keeping resources available for movement, repair, and stress response.

The Kidney decides how heavy the backpack needs to be for the entire journey — governing long-term reserve based on the body's constitutional assessment of endurance and future need.

Lipid panels reflect both processes simultaneously. A value that looks like excess from a population-risk perspective may reflect appropriate reserve from a constitutional perspective. The number alone cannot tell you which one it is. The patient's history, symptoms, and lived experience are part of that answer.

ORGAN TIME AND THE LIPID PANEL

Lipid panels are drawn fasting, in the early morning — which means they are collected during the Gallbladder Organ Time window (5–7 AM) or the Pericardium window (7–9 AM), depending on collection time. Both are periods of transition: the Gallbladder window represents the end of the overnight detoxification cycle and the beginning of bile production for the day's digestive demands. The Pericardium window represents the morning cardiovascular mobilization phase, when the body is ramping up for the day's output.

Morning fasting lipid values therefore reflect the body's storage and reserve state after overnight regulation — not how lipids are mobilized under the stress, emotional load, or physical demand of a full day. This matters particularly for triglycerides, which are sensitive to recent dietary intake, stress-induced cortisol spikes, and sleep quality in the days preceding the draw. A patient who slept poorly for three nights before a blood draw, or who was under significant emotional stress in the week prior, may show triglyceride values that reflect that acute state rather than their baseline metabolic pattern.

In clinical practice, I routinely ask patients about the week before a lipid draw — not because the standardized fasting protocol is wrong, but because a single morning value in the context of an atypical week is a less reliable data point than most reports acknowledge. Trends across multiple draws, collected under reasonably consistent conditions, tell a considerably more accurate story than any single panel.

The Liver's Organ Time window — 3 to 5 AM — is when hepatic lipid production, cholesterol synthesis, and hormonal clearance are most active. This is the window the body uses to prepare the day's lipid availability. A blood draw taken at 7 AM is capturing the output of that overnight production cycle. It is a useful snapshot. It does not capture how that lipid availability performs across the day's demands.

READING LIPIDS WITH CLARITY RATHER THAN FEAR

The most useful shift in reading a lipid panel is moving from the question "is this dangerous?" to "what is this body doing, and does it make sense given what this person is living?" The first question produces anxiety and often unnecessary intervention. The second produces understanding and, when intervention is genuinely needed, a more precise and appropriate one.

Western Medicine uses lipid values to estimate cardiovascular risk. That function is important and should not be dismissed. Chinese Medicine uses those same values to assess reserve, constitutional strategy, and the relationship between availability and demand. Together, they produce a picture that neither system produces alone.

Patients benefit when lipid trends are evaluated over time, in relation to inflammatory markers, sleep quality, stress load, hormonal state, and recovery capacity. A single measurement rarely conveys the full story. What it does is open a conversation — and the quality of that conversation depends entirely on whether the number is the end of the inquiry or the beginning of it.

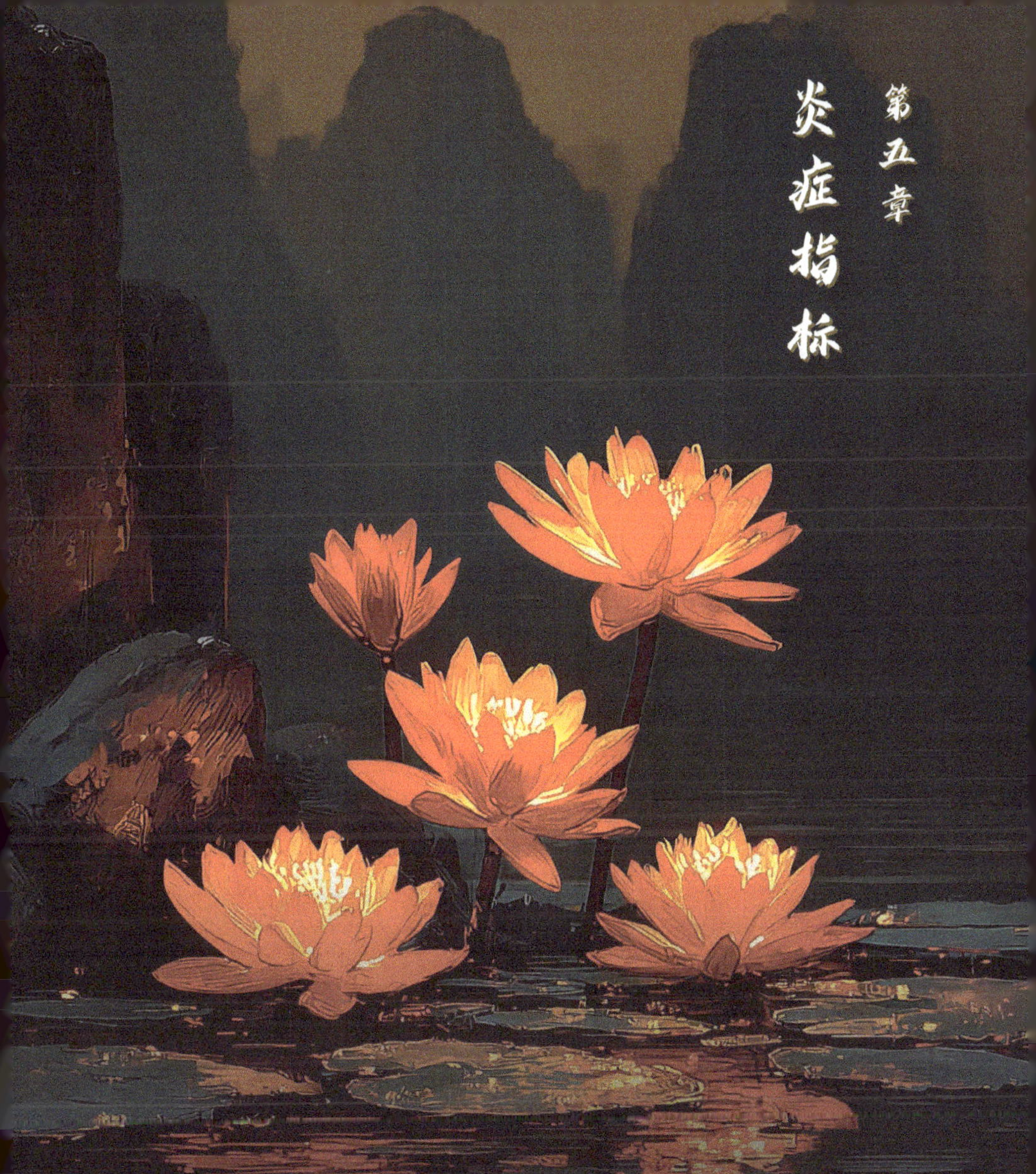

第五章

炎症指标

CHAPTER 5

Inflammatory Markers

PROTECTING, RESOLVING, OR LINGERING

Inflammatory Markers

PROTECTING, RESOLVING, OR LINGERING

Inflammation may be the most misunderstood word in modern healthcare. Not because it is poorly defined — the biology is well established — but because it has been flattened into a single category of pathology to be suppressed, rather than recognized as a biological process with distinct phases, distinct purposes, and distinct outcomes depending on whether it completes or stalls.

Patients come in having been told they "have inflammation" as though that phrase is a diagnosis. It is not. It is the beginning of a question. Inflammation that is actively protecting tissue is not the same as inflammation that resolved last month. Inflammation that peaks every afternoon at 4 PM and recedes by morning is not the same as inflammation that is constant. Inflammation that is driving a healing process is not the same as inflammation that has become the problem because the healing process cannot finish.

Both Western Medicine and Chinese Medicine recognize inflammation as meaningful. They differ in what they listen for — and in what they consider a satisfactory answer.

WHAT WESTERN MEDICINE MEASURES

Western inflammatory markers are calibrated to detect acute danger: active infection, autoimmune activity, significant tissue injury, or systemic disease requiring intervention. The three most commonly ordered are C-reactive protein (CRP), erythrocyte sedimentation rate (ESR), and ferritin.

C-Reactive Protein (CRP)

C-reactive protein is produced by the liver in response to inflammatory signaling. It rises quickly — within hours — when inflammation is present, and falls as inflammation resolves. Markedly elevated CRP levels prompt evaluation for infection, trauma, or active autoimmune disease. This is a well-designed early warning system for acute inflammatory events.

Its limitation is scope, not accuracy. CRP identifies that inflammation is present. It does not identify whether that inflammation is in its early protective phase or its chronic lingering phase. It does not record what time of day the marker is most elevated. It does not distinguish between inflammation driven by an acute event and inflammation driven by the cumulative weight of years of unresolved stress, poor sleep, and emotional load. The number is real. The context around it is what makes it interpretable.

Erythrocyte Sedimentation Rate (ESR)

Erythrocyte sedimentation rate measures how rapidly red blood cells settle in a test tube. When inflammatory proteins are present in the blood, it becomes more viscous and cells settle faster. ESR rises more slowly than CRP and reflects longer-standing or chronic inflammatory activity rather than acute events. A patient with persistently elevated ESR alongside a normal CRP is describing a slow-burning pattern — not an emergency, but not resolution either. That pattern deserves attention precisely because it is easy to overlook when nothing is dramatically abnormal.

Ferritin

Ferritin is described on most lab reports as an iron-storage protein, which it is. What is less often communicated is that ferritin also functions as an acute-phase reactant — it rises in response to inflammation and liver stress, independent of iron stores. An elevated ferritin in a patient with normal iron levels is not a storage problem. It is an inflammatory signal that the report's label has obscured. Elevated ferritin in the context of normal iron is one of the markers I have found most consistently correlated with chronic inflammatory load — particularly in patients whose CRP appears reassuringly normal because their inflammatory activity peaks outside the morning draw window.

WHAT CHINESE MEDICINE LISTENS FOR

Chinese Medicine does not view inflammation as a pathological intrusion. It views it as a phase in the body's healing cycle — necessary, purposeful, and designed to complete. The clinical question is not whether inflammation is occurring. It is whether the body has what it needs to finish the process.

When inflammation stalls — when it lingers beyond its protective phase, circling without resolution — Chinese Medicine interprets this as Stagnation: impaired circulation, insufficient nourishment, or depletion of the resources the body needs to complete its own repair. The cause may be physical: inadequate rest, nutritional deficiency, or a system so burdened by other demands that it cannot allocate enough to finish what it started. Or it may be emotional: unresolved grief, chronic frustration, or the kind of sustained low-grade stress that never quite reaches crisis but never fully releases either.

Inflammation is not the enemy. When read clearly, it is the body signaling what it needs in order for healing to complete.

This is a clinically significant distinction. Suppressing inflammation pharmacologically without addressing why it is not resolving on its own often produces temporary relief followed by recurrence. The body will keep signaling until the underlying condition that prevented resolution is addressed. Supporting circulation, nourishment, rest, and rhythm — giving the body what it needs to finish the process — is a different clinical strategy than quieting the signal.

八纲, Bā Gāng: The Eight Principles

The Ba Gang (八纲, Bā Gāng) is a classical Chinese Medicine diagnostic framework that organizes clinical findings into four pairs of opposites:

Yin and Yang — the fundamental balance of cooling/nourishing versus warming/activating

Excess and Deficiency — too much of something versus not enough

Heat and Cold — the thermal quality of the pattern

Interior and Exterior — whether the condition is on the surface or deep within the system

Applied to inflammation: Heat-Excess-Interior describes an acute infection with active fever and systemic involvement. Cold-Deficiency-Interior describes a chronic, low-grade inflammatory pattern in a depleted patient whose body cannot generate enough warmth and circulation to complete the healing cycle. Same word — inflammation — two completely different clinical pictures requiring two completely different responses. The Ba Gang is one of the tools that makes that distinction legible.

ORGAN TIME AND THE INFLAMMATORY CYCLE

Inflammation is not static across the day. It rises and falls in response to stress, activity, digestion, sleep, and emotional demand — and in many patients, it follows a consistent and recognizable pattern that the standard morning blood draw is poorly positioned to capture.

Using Organ Time, the afternoon inflammatory peak that many patients describe — joint stiffness, body aches, sensations of heat, histamine reactivity — falls within the Stomach window (3–5 PM). The Stomach governs digestive transformation and is closely tied to the body's processing of what has been taken in across the day, including food, stress, and environmental demand. Inflammatory activity that peaks in this window often has a digestive or dietary component — food sensitivities, incomplete digestion, or the cumulative metabolic load of a full day expressing itself as the body shifts from output toward repair.

The Lung window (5–7 PM) represents the body's transition into its surface-boundary and immune-regulation phase. Inflammatory symptoms that intensify in the early evening — respiratory sensitivity, skin reactivity, a sensation of heat moving to the surface — are often Lung-window presentations. The Lung governs the body's first-line immune response and its boundary with the external environment. When that system is strained, the late afternoon and early evening is when it tends to show.

A C-reactive protein (CRP) drawn at 8 AM in a fasting patient will often appear entirely normal in someone whose inflammatory activity peaks at 4 PM. The marker is real. The draw time missed it. Clinically, this mismatch between when a patient's inflammatory symptoms consistently occur and when their blood was collected, is one of the most common explanations for the experience of being told your labs are normal, this mismatch — between when a patient's inflammatory symptoms consistently occur and when their blood was collected — is one of the most common explanations for the experience of being told your labs are normal while your body is clearly telling a different story.

Inflammatory complaints that worsen at night — after the day's external demands have ended and the body turns its attention inward toward repair — are understood differently from those present upon waking. Nighttime aggravation, particularly in the Liver window (3–5 AM), often suggests that the body is struggling to complete its repair cycle during the hours specifically designated for that purpose. The effort is there. The resources to finish it are not.

INFLAMMATION THAT PROTECTS VERSUS INFLAMMATION THAT EXHAUSTS

The physician 孙思邈 (Sūn Sīmiǎo), one of the most revered clinicians in the history of Chinese Medicine, emphasized not only the treatment of acute illness but the cultivation of conditions that prevented the need for emergency intervention. Urgent care and long-term health were understood as part of the same continuum — and the physician's responsibility extended across both ends of it.

That framing remains clinically sound. Western Medicine

excels at identifying when inflammation has crossed into acute danger and intervening decisively. Chinese Medicine listens for the patterns that precede that crossing — the persistent low-grade elevation, the incomplete resolution, the marker that keeps returning to the same borderline value because the body cannot finish what it keeps trying to start.

Together, these perspectives allow a more complete reading of inflammatory markers than either system produces alone. Not every elevated CRP requires aggressive intervention. Not every normal CRP means the inflammatory picture is clear. The marker is one data point. When, how consistently, in what context, and alongside what symptoms it appears — those are the questions that turn a number into a clinical understanding.

When inflammation is read clearly, it is not a threat. It is a signal. And signals, when properly interpreted, tell you exactly what the body needs in order to heal.

One dimension of that signal that laboratory panels rarely capture is the emotional one. Chronic anger, sustained grief, and prolonged fear each produce measurable inflammatory activity — elevated CRP, elevated cortisol, suppressed immune coordination. In Chinese Medicine, these are not metaphors. They are physiological patterns with organ-system involvement. The full mapping of the seven emotions to their hormonal and inflammatory signatures is covered in Chapter 6, where the relationship between emotional experience and laboratory findings is developed in clinical detail.

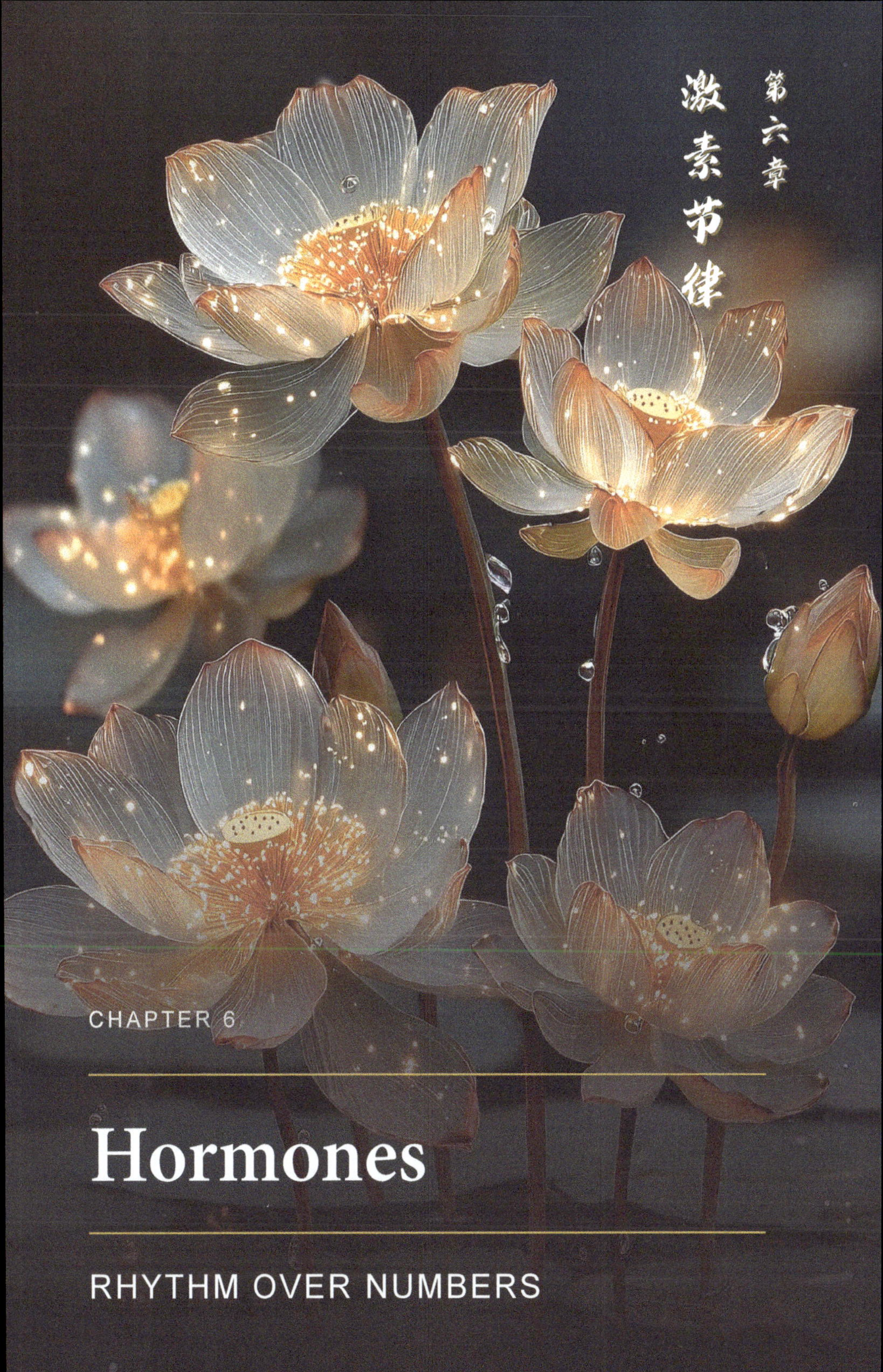

第六章

激素节律

CHAPTER 6

Hormones

RHYTHM OVER NUMBERS

Hormones

RHYTHM OVER NUMBERS

Hormones are the body's internal communication system. They are how tissues know what time it is, what the body is being asked to do, and what resources are available to do it. Released by glands, carried through the bloodstream, and received by target tissues across the body, hormones coordinate virtually every function that matters: growth, metabolism, mood, immunity, reproduction, sleep, repair, and recovery.

The critical word in that list is coordinate. Hormones do not simply exist in the blood at a concentration. They signal. They sequence. They rise at the right moment and fall when their work is done — and the difference between a hormone functioning well and the same hormone producing symptoms is often not its quantity but its timing.

This is the conversation that most hormone panels do not have. They measure how much. They rarely address when, in what sequence, or whether the signal is arriving at the tissue that needs it with the right strength at the right hour. A single morning blood value captures one frame of a film that runs continuously. Understanding what that frame is showing — and what it cannot show — is what this chapter is about.

Hormone tests do not define the body.
They describe a moment within its rhythm.

WHAT WESTERN MEDICINE EVALUATES

Western Medicine evaluates hormones primarily to identify deficiency, excess, or structural disease of the endocrine glands. Thyroid panels, cortisol testing, insulin measures, and reproductive hormone values are essential for diagnosing conditions such as hypothyroidism, adrenal insufficiency, diabetes, or reproductive dysfunction. When production falls outside safe limits — severe thyroid imbalance, adrenal failure, uncontrolled blood sugar — prompt intervention is appropriate and often necessary. In these situations, numbers matter enormously. Identifying gland failure or extreme dysfunction is lifesaving work.

Where this form of evaluation becomes less informative is in the space between failure and optimal function. A hormone may be produced in adequate quantity yet released at the wrong hour, converted inefficiently into its active form, or poorly received by the tissues it is meant to serve. In these cases, laboratory values appear reassuring while the patient continues to feel unwell. The gland is not failing. The signal is not arriving correctly. Those are two different problems with two different solutions, and a single reference-range comparison cannot distinguish between them.

HORMONES AS SEQUENCES, NOT SNAPSHOTS

The Thyroid — A Production and Conversion Story

The thyroid is often discussed as a single system, but it functions as a sequence. Thyroid-stimulating hormone (TSH) is produced by the pituitary gland to signal the thyroid to produce thyroxine (T4) — a reserve form of thyroid hormone. T4 must then be converted in peripheral tissues, primarily the liver and kidneys, into triiodothyronine (T3) — the active form that actually drives metabolism, temperature regulation, and cognitive speed.

A patient may have TSH, free T4, and free T3 values all within reference range and still experience cold sensitivity, fatigue, weight changes, or slowed thinking. From a Chinese Medicine perspective, this reflects a problem of transformation or delivery rather than production. The gland is doing its job. The conversion is where the efficiency has declined. Liver strain, nutritional depletion, chronic stress, or hormonal burden can all impair the T4-to-T3 conversion step without producing values that cross a diagnostic threshold.

This is one of the patterns I encounter most consistently in practice: a patient with thyroid symptoms and a "normal" thyroid panel, whose free T3 sits at the lower end of the reference range while free T4 appears adequate. The production is fine. The delivery is not. That distinction does not appear in a simple TSH result.

Cortisol — The Timing Hormone

Cortisol is not simply a stress hormone. It is a timing hormone. Its primary job is to signal the body what time of day it is and what is required of it at that moment. It should rise sharply in the hour after waking — the cortisol awakening response — reaching its peak between 8 and 10 AM, then declining gradually across the day to its lowest point around midnight.

Many patients experience the precise opposite: difficulty waking, low energy in the morning, an afternoon that feels manageable only with caffeine, and then a second wind that arrives inconveniently around 10 PM when the body should be preparing for sleep. This is a cortisol rhythm problem, not a cortisol quantity problem. A single morning draw — which is the standard — may show a cortisol value within reference range while completely missing the fact that the curve is inverted. The number looks fine. The pattern does not.

Reproductive Hormones — Estrogen, Progesterone, and Testosterone

Estradiol and progesterone vary enormously across the menstrual cycle. A value of 40 pg/mL is appropriate in the follicular phase and insufficient in the mid-luteal phase. Drawing these values without documenting cycle day and time of collection produces numbers that are technically accurate and clinically uninterpretable. Yet cycle day is routinely not recorded on lab requisitions, and time of collection almost never is.

Testosterone follows a clear diurnal pattern in both men and women, typically 25 to 50 percent higher in the early morning than in the late afternoon. A testosterone value drawn at 4 PM will look meaningfully different from one drawn at 8 AM in the same individual on the same day. For patients with borderline values, the hour of collection can determine whether the result prompts a clinical conversation or produces a reassuring normal. Same patient. Same physiology. Different hour.

Hormone D3 — The Biliary Bone Matrix Hormone

What is commonly labeled Vitamin D3 on laboratory reports is not a vitamin. It is a hormone — synthesized in the skin from ultraviolet light exposure as cholecalciferol, converted by the liver into 25-hydroxyvitamin D (the form most labs actually measure and report), and activated by the kidneys into 1,25-dihydroxyvitamin D (calcitriol) — the form that functions through nuclear receptors to regulate gene expression across multiple organ systems. A substance manufactured by the body from sunlight, requiring multi-organ conversion before activation, and governing calcium metabolism, immune regulation, and inflammatory signaling through receptor-mediated pathways is, by every pharmacological definition, a hormone.

The name of this section — Biliary Bone Matrix Hormone — is written in the cinematic language the primer introduced. Biliary points to the Liver-Gallbladder scene: bile production, fat emulsification, hormonal conversion, the smooth flow of material through the body's processing pathways. Bone points to the Kidney scene: the deep structural reserve, the mineral economy, the constitutional layer where what the body has built over a lifetime is held. Matrix is what ties them together — the living tissue field through which this hormone moves, is activated, and does its work.

One hormone, two scenes, one matrix. The Western biochemistry describes the conversion pathway. The TCM character set describes the terrain that conversion moves through. Neither is the whole picture on its own.

In Chinese Medicine, Hormone D3's production and conversion pathway runs directly through the Liver and Gallbladder — the biliary matrix that governs fat metabolism, hormonal conversion, and mineral distribution — and into the Kidney, which governs bone, marrow, and the body's constitutional reserve. Low Hormone D3 in a patient with compromised Liver or Gallbladder function is not a simple supplementation problem. It is a conversion problem. The precursor may be adequate. The pathway to activation is where the deficit lives.

The clinical consequences of mislabeling it have been significant. Because it is categorized as a vitamin, Hormone D3 is routinely under-ordered, under-interpreted, and disconnected from the hormonal and biliary context where it actually belongs.

CHINESE MEDICINE — HORMONES AS RHYTHM AND COORDINATION

Chinese Medicine has always understood physiology as rhythmic. The body is not a collection of static levels to be maintained — it is a sequence of processes that rise and fall in coordination with each other and with the time of day. Hormonal health, from this perspective, depends less on absolute quantity and more on appropriate timing, smooth transformation, and the functional relationship between the systems involved in producing, converting, and receiving hormonal signals.

The Ba Gang (八纲, Bā Gāng) framework introduced in the previous chapter applies directly here. A hormonal pattern that reads as Yin Deficiency — insufficient cooling, nourishing, and containing capacity — produces a recognizable cluster: afternoon fatigue, night sweats, insomnia with difficulty staying asleep, heat sensations in the evening, emotional volatility, and a quality of depletion that rest does not fully resolve. A hormonal pattern that reads as Yang Deficiency — insufficient warmth, mobilization, and activating capacity — produces a different cluster: cold sensitivity, morning fatigue that does not lift easily, low motivation, slow metabolism, and a quality of heaviness that is present even after adequate sleep.

These are not diagnoses from a single laboratory value. They are patterns observed across the full clinical picture — including the time of day when symptoms are most present, which organ systems are involved, and what the patient's lived experience is telling us that the numbers are not.

Three Organ Patterns in Hormonal Imbalance

Liver-related hormonal patterns often show up as irritability, tension, headaches, digestive discomfort, or difficulty winding down at night. The Liver governs smooth movement of Qi and Blood — when it is strained, hormonal fluctuation becomes erratic and emotional regulation suffers alongside it.

Spleen-related hormonal patterns often appear as afternoon fatigue, brain fog, bloating, or feeling drained after meals. The Spleen governs transformation and transportation — when it is weak, the conversion of nutrients into hormonal precursors becomes inefficient and energy output becomes unreliable.

Kidney-related hormonal patterns often involve poor sleep, early-morning exhaustion, low resilience, cold sensitivity, or feeling depleted despite adequate rest. The Kidney governs long-term reserve — the deep constitutional capacity that hormonal production draws upon over time. When Kidney Jing (精, Jīng) is depleted, hormonal output may remain technically within range while the body's ability to sustain that output is quietly failing.

THE SEVEN EMOTIONS — 七情 (QĪ QÍNG)

In Chinese Medicine there are seven emotions: fear, fright, anger, sadness, melancholy, worry, and joy. I have come to realize that these are not just psychological categories, they are physiological events. Each emotion, when experienced acutely, is a normal and healthy expression of the body's response to life. When sustained chronically or expressed without resolution, each emotion also becomes a clinical pattern — one that produces measurable changes in hormone levels, inflammatory markers, and organ function, if you know how to look.

In clinical practice, I often describe cortisol to my patients as liquid fear. It is the most tangible example and how I could relate their emotional response to what happens in the body. Cortisol is measured in the blood as a hormone — the body's chemical translation of a perceived threat into physiological readiness. But cortisol is not the only emotion the body feels when it comes to the production of hormones. As this observation refined itself across years of patient encounters, it became clear that each of the seven emotions has a biochemical signature, and that signature shows up in laboratory panels, directly or indirectly. Most clinicians read these panels without taking into account the objective data of the examination process.

Understanding the emotional-hormonal relationship does not require abandoning Western medicine's precision. It requires taking into account complete clinical data and putting it into the patient's perspective as they go through their lived experience. Especially their history and whatever complaints they have named as the priority at that moment in their life.

THE SEVEN EMOTIONS - 七情 (QĪ QÍNG)

HOW TO USE THIS CHART

Each entry maps one of the Seven Emotions to its governing organ, its Five Element identity — including the actual physical movement of that emotion through the body as described in the Huangdi Neijing and Nanjing, its taste, and its thermal nature — and its hormonal signature in the biomedical system.

The liquid name beneath each elevated hormone translates that emotion into its measurable chemical form. The flavors and directions describe the movement of the emotion itself — what the body is doing — not the therapeutic correction. Bitter descending is what Fire needs to correct itself; Fire's own movement is upward and outward, and its flavor is pungent.

The Liver is the seat of all emotion. Every emotion described here begins with the Liver — either expressing through it, overacting on another organ through it, or being compressed within it.

WATER - KIDNEY & BLADDER

Cold **Salty & Bitter** **Sinking ↓ Inward**

Non-movement / Paralysis

Healthy movement: downward and inward — storing, consolidating, descending to root. Taste: salty — softening and sinking, the most inward and downward of all flavors. Bitter is secondary — fear depletes over time. Temperature: cold — most Yin, most inward. Fear softens, settles, and creates non-movement — a kind of paralysis. Cold like an iceberg, sinking downward and inward.

Fear

恐 (Kǒng)

Chronic / Inward — Yin expression of Water

WATER

Kidney

Cold **Sinking ↓ Inward** **Salty & Bitter**

Yin Expression

ELEVATED	SUPPRESSED	IN LABS
Cortisol	DHEA	↑ Cortisol
	Testosterone	↓ DHEA ratio
	Progesterone	↓ Testosterone
	Growth hormone	

liquid fear

cold, sinking, softening — the body's chemistry of paralysis and sustained threat

WOOD — LIVER & GALLBLADDER: THE SEAT OF ALL EMOTION

Warm → Hot | **Sour / Pungent / Sour & Bitter**

Variable by Expression | **Liver Governs All Emotion**

The Liver is the seat of all emotion. Every emotion is generated by it. Healthy movement: is upward — smooth, free-flowing, like a tree growing toward light. Taste: sweet — building then releasing. Fright is like Metal Yang energy (ie: spicy) suddenly overacting on the Liver, making the Gallbladder react into sudden Yang expression. Constraint is the sour compression contracting inward. This leads to anger which friction and compression becomes fire expression. Joy is Wood over-supplying Fire energy — the Liver flooding the Heart with Blood.

Fright

驚 (Jīng)

Acute / Outward — Metal Yang overacting on Liver - Gallbladder consolidates via GB 25 (首門)

WOOD

Gallbladder

Hot Spike | **Exploding ↗ Outward** | **Pungent / Spicy**

Yang Spike

ELEVATED	SUPPRESSED	IN LABS
Adrenaline	Oxytocin	↑ Adrenaline
Norepinephrine	Serotonin	↓ DHEA post-event
Acute cortisol	DHEA	Cortisol spike then
	(post-shock drop)	crash

liquid fright

a sudden stab — pungent at its zenith, spicy and hot; the Liver's Yin nature driven instantly outward

Constraint / Frustration

鬱 (Yù)

Liver Qi Stagnation: sour compression descending to its bottom — Yin expression of Wood

WOOD

Liver

Hold | Downward ↓ Inward | Sour & Bitter

Yin Expression

ELEVATED	SUPPRESSED	IN LABS
Prolactin	Dopamine	↓ Dopamine
	Serotonin	↓ T3
	Progesterone	↓ Progesterone
	Testosterone	↑ Prolactin
	Thyroid T3 (Qi not converting from Blood)	

liquid frustration

sour compression moving downward and inward — bitter emerges as bile releases at the nadir of the held movement

Anger

怒 (Nù)

Liver Fire: compression becomes friction, friction becomes flame — Yang expression of Wood

WOOD

Liver

Warm → Hot | Upward ↑ Outward → | Pungent

Yang Expression

ELEVATED	SUPPRESSED	IN LABS
Testosterone	Serotonin	↑ CRP
Adrenaline	Oxytocin	↑ Testosterone
CRP	Progesterone	↑ Liver enzymes
Estrogen (excess)		↓ Serotonin

liquid anger

pungent — upward and outward — Wood's compressed energy breaking into flame

FIRE — HEART & PERICARDIUM

Hot **Pungent** **Upward & Outward ↗**

Wood Feeding Fire

Fire's actual movement is upward and outward — its flavor expression is pungent. Bitter is what Fire needs to descend and correct excess, not what Fire does. The Liver stores Blood and the Heart commands Blood. When Wood overfeeds Fire — too much Blood flooding the Heart — the Shen comes to the face. Spontaneous laughter or laughing at things that are not funny (ie: Gallows Syndrome).

Joy / Mania

喜 (Xǐ)

Wood feeding Fire: Shen coming to the face: Gallows Syndrome

FIRE

Heart

Hot **Upward ↑ Outward ↗** **Pungent**

Yang Expression

ELEVATED	SUPPRESSED	IN LABS
Dopamine	Norepinephrine (post-peak)	↑ Dopamine
Serotonin	DHEA (after excess)	↑ Serotonin
Oxytocin		Post-peak depletion
Estrogen (briefly)		

liquid joy

pungent — upward and outward — Liver flooding the Heart with Blood, Shen expressing through the face

EARTH — SPLEEN & STOMACH

Neutral **Bland** **Circling / Holding ↻**

Liver Overacting on Spleen

The Liver overacts on the Spleen, like a plane in a holding pattern, the thoughts roll through the Spleen without landing — circling waiting for a place to be directed in order to complete its journey to clarity. Taste: bland — not sweet. Sweet is Earth's healthy expression; bland is what emerges when the Spleen's transformation is burdened and exhausted, it becomes flat. The metabolic cost of a mind that cannot stop circling falls entirely on the Spleen.

Worry / Overthinking

思 (Sī)

Liver overacting on Spleen: thoughts in a holding pattern — Yin expression of Earth

EARTH

Spleen

Neutral | Circling / Holding ↻ | Bland

Yin Expresion

ELEVATED	SUPPRESSED	IN LABS
Insulin	DHEA	↑ Insulin
Prolactin	Growth hormone	↓ DHEA
	Serotonin	↓ Growth hormone
	Testosterone	Flat energy curve

liquid worry

the metabolic cost of thoughts that circle without landing — Liver holding the Spleen in pattern

METAL — LUNG & LARGE INTESTINE

Sour | **Cool → Cold** | **Contracting & Inward**

Liver Counteracting Lung

The Liver counteracts the Lung, creating a sour, compressing, inward movement — like squeezing a sponge. The water comes to the surface: this is weeping and crying. The character for Sadness (悲) shows the heart going back and sinking into the body — the person sinks, head drops, spine arches as the compression completes. This is the Yang within Yin expression of Metal — active release through inward compression. Once the fluid is expressed and the Qi exits, the body settles into inactivity — Depression / Melancholy, the Yin within Yin. The dispersing function has failed entirely. Cool becoming cold. The sponge has been squeezed dry.

Sadness / Grief

悲 (Bēi)

Active, Inward: Weeping, crying — Yang within Yin expression of Metal

METAL

Lung

Cool | Contracting & Inward | Sour

Yang Within Yin

ELEVATED	SUPPRESSED	IN LABS
Prolactin	Serotonin	↑ Prolactin
CRP	Oxytocin	↓ Serotonin
	Testosterone	↓ Oxytocin

liquid sadness

sour contracting inward — the Liver squeezing the Lung like a sponge, fluid rising to the surface as tears

Depression / Melancholy

憂 (Yōu)

Inward, still: fluid expressed, Qi gone, body settles — Yin within Yin expression of Metal

METAL

Lung

Cold | Inward & Deep ↓ | Sour — Collapsed

Yin within Yin

ELEVATED	SUPPRESSED	IN LABS
(minimal — the sponge has been squeezed dry, nothing left to release)	Dopamine Serotonin Testosterone Thyroid T3 DHEA Estrogen Growth hormone	↓ Dopamine ↓ T3 ↓ Testosterone ↓ DHEA ↓ Suppressed across the panel

liquid melancholy

the body still — cool becoming cold — the sour movement exhausted and collapsed

APPENDIX — HORMONAL MATERIA MEDICA

A Classical Chinese Classification of the Body's Chemical Messengers

In Chinese Medicine, every herb is described by its flavor, thermal nature, direction of movement, and organ affinity — properties that explain not only what the herb does, but why it goes where it goes and which part of the body it speaks to. Every hormone below is classified by that same lens. The liquid name for each hormone is drawn directly from the Seven Emotions — so the reader need only know the emotion to understand the chemistry. Cortisol is Liquid Fear. Adrenaline is Liquid Fright. The language stays consistent from the chart to the lab report.

Hormone & Liquid Name	Flavor & Temp	Direction of Movement	Organ Affinity	What It Means Emotionally
Cortisol *Liquid Fear*	Salty Cold	Sinking ↓ Inward	Kidney	The chemical form of a body under sustained threat. Cold and descending, it suppresses every warming and building hormone in service of survival. When cortisol stays high, the body is chemically frozen in fear — even when the original threat is long gone.
Adrenaline *Liquid Fright*	Pungent/ Spicy Hot	Exploding ↑ ↗ Outward	Gallbladder	The body's sudden startle made chemical — designed to fire fast and clear fast. When it cannot clear, it consolidates into Fear via the Gallbladder-Kidney pathway. The difference between fright and fear is whether this chemistry was allowed to complete its movement.

Hormone & Liquid Name	Flavor & Temp	Direction of Movement	Organ Affinity	What It Means Emotionally
Norepinephrine ***Liquid Fright*** (directed)	Pungent *Hot*	Upward ↑ Directed	Heart / Gallbladder	The directional component of fright — where adrenaline explodes outward, norepinephrine aims. Together they form the chemistry of acute shock. Depleted in both Joy excess and Depression. When it is low, the body cannot direct its own attention or response.
Testosterone ***Liquid Anger***	Pungent *Warm*	Upward ↑ Outward →	Gallbladder/ Liver/ Kidney Axis	Wood's Yang energy rising from Water's root — the warmth of mobilizing, asserting, and expressing. In anger it is the heat breaking through. In fear and constraint it is the first thing suppressed, because survival does not need expression, it needs containment.
Prolactin ***Liquid Frustration***	Sour → Bitter *Neutral –Cool*	Inward / Arrested ↔	Liver	What the body makes when substance accumulates faster than it can move. Elevated in constraint, sadness, and worry — three emotions defined by something that cannot complete its movement. It is the chemistry of engorgement without release, of presence without expression, of holding what was meant to be given.

Hormone & Liquid Name	Flavor & Temp	Direction of Movement	Organ Affinity	What It Means Emotionally
Dopamine *Liquid Joy*	Bitter *Warm – Hot*	Upward ↑ Outward ↗	Heart	The spark that starts movement — motivation, initiation, reward. In balance: joy. In excess: mania. Depleted in constraint and depression. When a patient says "I know what I need to do but I cannot make myself do it," this is often the missing chemistry of joy withdrawn from the body.
Serotonin *Liquid Joy* (sustained)	Sweet *Neutral –Warm*	Centering / Distributing	Heart	The quiet sustaining of joy — Earth nourishing Fire. Not excitement, but ease. The sense that things are manageable. Depleted in nearly every chronic emotion. Its absence is rarely dramatic — it is the slow dimming of what used to feel ordinary and fine.
Oxytocin *Liquid Joy*	Sweet *Warm*	Outward → Connecting	Heart	The relational dimension of joy — the warmth of the Heart opening toward another person. Depleted by fright, anger, and sadness. Its absence is often the quiet signal of isolation the lab panel never names. A patient who has lost the ability to feel close to others has often lost this first.

Hormone & Liquid Name	Flavor & Temp	Direction of Movement	Organ Affinity	What It Means Emotionally
DHEA *Liquid Joy* (precursor of all Yang)	Sweet–Pungent *Warm*	Upward ↑ Rising potential	Heart	The reserve beneath joy. Where growth hormone expresses vitality in the moment, DHEA is the stored capacity that makes joy sustainable over a lifetime — the precursor that feeds every Yang hormone and the substrate every emotion draws from. Depleted across all Seven Emotions when they become chronic. Its ratio to cortisol is one of the most honest readings in the panel: how long has this body been under pressure, and how much of its joy remains available?
Insulin *Liquid Worry*	Sweet *Neutral*	Inward ↓ Into cells	Spleen / Stomach	Earth's transformation made chemical — moving food into fuel. In worry and overthinking, the Spleen is overburdened and insulin rises with it. The body pays a metabolic price for a mind that will not rest. Blood sugar instability is often a Spleen story written in the body's chemistry.
Progesterone *Liquid Worry* (Yin containment)	Sweet Cool	Inward ↓ Containing	Kidney / Liver	What the body makes when the system turns inward to protect. Elevated in worry, rumination, and preservation — the mind circling the same concern, the body guarding itself against loss. It is the chemistry of holding on past the moment of need, of nourishment that has become heaviness, of stillness that has forgotten how to move.

Hormone & Liquid Name	Flavor & Temp	Direction of Movement	Organ Affinity	What It Means Emotionally
Thyroid T3 ***Liquid Frustration*** (conversion blocked)	Bitter–Sour *Warm*	Downward ↓ Inward ↓	Lung / Large Intestine	The active form of metabolic expression — what drives temperature, speed, and cognitive clarity. Depleted in constraint and depression: not a production problem, a conversion problem. The body has the raw material but cannot transform it — the same pattern as Liver Qi Stagnation expressed in the thyroid axis.
Growth Hormone ***Liquid Joy***	Sweet *Warm*	Upward ↑	Heart	The chemistry of rising into life. Released in deep sleep and childhood, it lifts the body into growth and the spirit into play — the hormone of laughter, vitality, and recovery. When pushed beyond its natural cycle through stress, overtraining, or outside sources, that same rising can turn fierce and aggressive. Joy is its nature; fury is what it becomes when it rises without rest beneath it.

Flavor (味, wèi), temperature (性, xìng), and direction of movement (升降浮沉 shēng jiàng fú chén) are assigned according to the classical Chinese Medicine materia medica framework. Liquid names are drawn directly from the Seven Emotions (七情, Qī Qíng) so that every hormone in this table maps back to the same emotional vocabulary used throughout this book. These classifications describe functional patterns based on physiological mechanisms.

Years of clinical practice have made one thing consistently clear for me: patients experiencing chronic fear, the emotion that affects the Kidneys, present with elevated cortisol, suppressed DHEA, and testosterone. Again, this is why I gave Cortisol the name liquid fear — the body's sustained chemical translation of perceived threat. When it stays elevated, everything else is suppressed in service of survival.

Now lets look at the other emotions. For example, sadness or grief, which is the Lung's outward Yang within Yin expression. Patients may show elevated prolactin and suppressed serotonin as well as oxytocin: the hormonal picture of a body expressing loss. Patients in the quieter, inward Yin within Yin Lung state — depression, melancholy, somberness, withdrawal — show suppression across nearly the entire panel: dopamine, T3, testosterone, DHEA, and estrogen. The body has stopped expressing. Patients experiencing Liver Qi Stagnation — the constraint and frustration that precedes anger — may show low dopamine, low T3, low progesterone, and elevated prolactin: things held, not converting, not flowing. The Blood is present, and the Qi (energy flow) is not yet released. When the stagnation finally breaks into Liver Fire — anger expressed — CRP rises, testosterone spikes, and the inflammatory markers that were quietly building finally show up on the panel.

What seems to be coincidences are not, once you understand that from a Chinese medicine perspective the seven emotions can be biomedically mapped. They are the body speaking its emotional history in the language of biochemis-

The blood test does not lie. It tells you exactly what the body has been living. The question is whether anyone in the room is trained to hear it.

try. The numbers on the report are not separate from the life that produced them.

Emotions leave a biochemical record. That record is often already in your blood work, waiting to be read correctly.

ORGAN TIME AND THE HORMONE PANEL

Most hormone panels are drawn in the early morning — which captures the body in its overnight storage and baseline regulation state. For cortisol, this is appropriate because the morning peak is the most clinically informative point in its cycle. For testosterone, the morning draw captures the daily high, which is the correct window for assessment. For thyroid markers, TSH peaks around midnight to 2 AM and reaches its daily low in the mid-afternoon — meaning an afternoon TSH draw can appear meaningfully lower than a morning draw in the same patient, a variation that matters when values are borderline.

Using Organ Time, the morning draw window falls across the Gallbladder period (5–7 AM) and the Pericardium period (7–9 AM). The Gallbladder window is when bile production activates and the liver's overnight hormonal clearance is completing — directly relevant to Hormone D3 conversion and sex hormone metabolism, both of which depend on hepatic and biliary function. The Pericardium window, peak cardiovascular mobilization time, is when testosterone is highest and cortisol is approaching its morning peak. Drawing hormone panels in this window captures the body at its most hormonally active and outwardly mobilized state.

What the morning draw does not capture is the afternoon and evening hormonal picture — when cortisol should be low, when insulin sensitivity has declined, when the body is managing the transition from output to repair. The patient whose cortisol is normal at 8 AM and elevated at 10 PM, whose testosterone is adequate in the morning and functionally insufficient by late afternoon, whose Hormone D3 conversion is impaired by a Liver system under strain — that patient's morning panel may show nothing remarkable. Their body is telling a different story at a different hour.

When symptoms consistently appear at certain times of day, they are not random. They are the body's hormonal rhythm expressing itself — and the time of day when that expression is loudest is rarely the time the blood was drawn.

WHEN THE RHYTHM IS RESTORED

Western Medicine excels at identifying endocrine disease — when a gland is failing, when production has crossed into dangerous territory, when medical intervention is required. That capacity is essential and should not be minimized.

Chinese Medicine focuses on restoring rhythm — how signals rise and fall across the day, how well the body transitions between activity and rest, how internal systems support one another's function over time. Rather than waiting for failure, it attends to strain, mistiming, and depletion before they accumulate into pathology.

Together, these perspectives explain one of the most common experiences in clinical practice: a patient who feels consistently unwell despite hormone panels that return within normal range. The body is frequently ahead of the laboratory — beginning to recover before values shift, or beginning to decline before values flag. Biochemical change — measurable shifts in hormone levels, receptors, or downstream markers — often lags behind functional change in both directions. Better sleep, steadier energy, improved mood, and clearer thinking may appear weeks before the numbers move. Declining function may be experienced for months before a value crosses a threshold.

Hormones are not switches. They are messengers moving through time, in sequence, in rhythm. When that rhythm is supported — through sleep, nourishment, timing-conscious clinical decisions, and attention to the pattern rather than only the number — the body regains coordination. That is when symptoms ease. The numbers often follow. But they are rarely the first sign that something has changed.

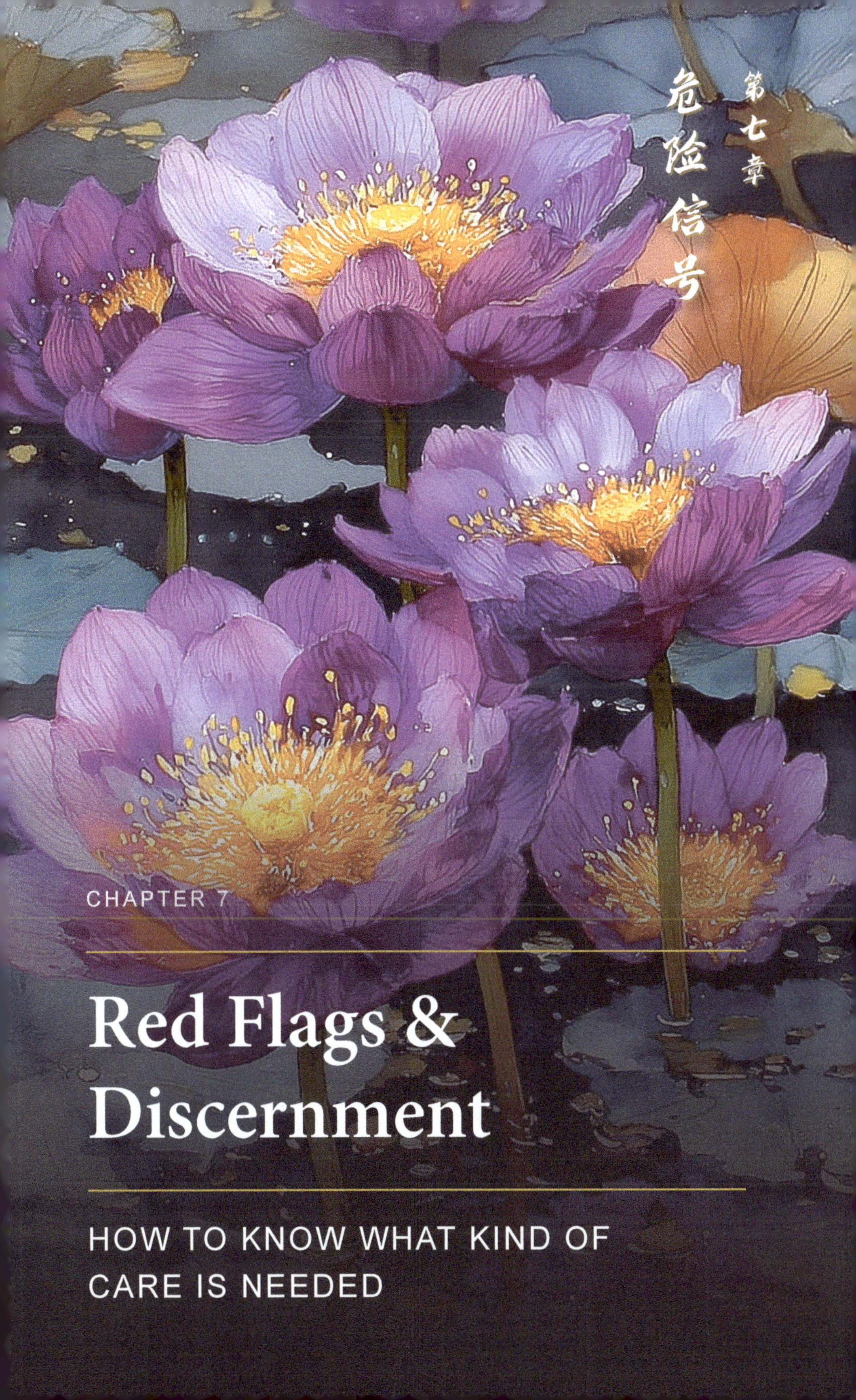

第七章
危险信号

CHAPTER 7

Red Flags & Discernment

HOW TO KNOW WHAT KIND OF CARE IS NEEDED

Red Flags & Discernment

HOW TO KNOW WHAT KIND OF CARE IS NEEDED

Discernment is one of the most undervalued clinical skills a patient can develop — and one of the least taught. It is the capacity to know when reassurance is appropriate and when deeper inquiry or immediate action is required. Without it, patients tend toward one of two equally unhelpful positions: dismissing symptoms that deserve attention, or escalating concern over findings that are being managed well. Modern healthcare, it must be said, often contributes to both problems simultaneously.

This chapter exists to restore proportion.

Red flags are not a modern invention. They did not arrive with laboratory medicine. They emerged across every medical tradition, in every era, from the same clinical necessity: a physician needs to be able to answer one question quickly and accurately. What level of response does this condition require right now? The tools for answering that question differ between traditions. The question itself does not.

WHERE RED FLAGS COME FROM

In Chinese medical history, the differentiation between emergency, urgent, acute, subacute, and chronic care has existed for over two thousand years. During the Warring States period, physicians were already distinguishing conditions that required immediate intervention from those that allowed time for observation and graduated response. This was not academic categorization. In an era of epidemic disease and military conflict, the ability to make that distinction quickly was the difference between a patient surviving and not.

张仲景 (Zhāng Zhòngjing), whose work during the Han dynasty addressed acute and epidemic conditions with a precision that remains clinically relevant today, developed formulas that were not gentle tonics. They were decisive, time-sensitive interventions designed to interrupt dangerous progression — the equivalent, in his era, of what we would now call emergency medicine. His work is still studied because the clinical logic is sound: recognize the pattern, assess the urgency, respond with appropriate force and appropriate restraint.

Centuries later, 孙思邈 (Sūn Sīmiǎo) expanded this framework beyond the emergency room of classical medicine. He emphasized not only the identification of acute danger but discernment across the full arc of illness — from the moment of crisis through recovery, rehabilitation, and the cultivation of conditions that prevented the next crisis. He understood something that is easy to lose in a system calibrated for acute intervention: over-treating a stable condition can be as harmful as under-treating an emergency. Both are failures of discernment.

Western Medicine developed along a parallel path. As anatomy, surgery, and laboratory diagnostics advanced, red flags became associated with findings that signaled immediate structural danger: hemorrhage, organ failure, infection, rapidly progressing disease. The goal was stabilization and survival. That goal is still the right one when the situation calls for it.

THE SPECTRUM OF CARE — BOTH SYSTEMS RECOGNIZE IT

Across both traditions, clinical response functions along a spectrum. What differs is not whether these categories exist, but how each system identifies when a patient has moved from one to the next.

The Spectrum of Care

Emergency Care — *Immediate threat to life or organ integrity. This is not a conversation. It is an intervention.*

Urgent Care — *Rapid progression that requires timely intervention before the window for effective response closes.*

Acute Care — *Active disease requiring focused treatment. The situation is serious but not immediately life-threatening.*

Subacute Care — *Incomplete recovery or lingering dysfunction. The crisis has passed but restoration has not been achieved.*

Chronic Care — *Long-standing patterns requiring sustained support. Not an emergency — but not something to ignore simply because the numbers are stable.*

Western Red Flags — When the Numbers Demand Action

In Western Medicine, a red flag is a finding that suggests immediate danger, rapid deterioration, or risk of irreversible harm. Profoundly abnormal electrolytes, rapidly rising kidney markers, severe anemia, markedly elevated liver enzymes, or inflammatory markers consistent with acute infection or autoimmune flare — these findings require prompt response, and in those situations, reassurance would be inappropriate.

The hemoglobin threshold for transfusion is a clean example. When hemoglobin falls below approximately 7 g/dL, the body's oxygen delivery capacity is compromised to a degree that threatens organ function. Transfusion is indicated. This is not a gray area. Western Medicine is designed for exactly this moment, and it handles it well.

These are true red flags. They signal collapse, not strain. They warrant the urgency they receive.

Chinese Medicine Red Flags – When the Pattern Demands Action

Chinese Medicine also recognizes emergencies – and has always included active emergency and urgent care within its framework. This point is worth stating clearly because it is frequently misunderstood. Chinese Medicine is not a system that waits patiently while a patient deteriorates, deferring to Western Medicine once things become serious. It has its own emergency medicine, its own urgent care protocols, and its own interventions for acute and life-threatening conditions.

Acute epidemic conditions – what classical texts described as 热毒 (Rè Dú, Heat Toxin) – include presentations we now recognize as severe bacterial or viral infections: high fever, rapid systemic involvement, inflammation, swelling, and the potential for collapse. These require immediate intervention. Modern Chinese hospitals treat emergency trauma alongside surgery with 云南白药 (Yúnnán Báiyào) to control bleeding, acute burns with topical formulations such as 三黄膏 (Sān Huáng Gāo, Three Yellow Ointment), and severe infections with classical formulas calibrated to the presentation. These are not passive interventions. They are precisely timed, precisely dosed, and directed at interrupting dangerous progression — which is exactly what emergency medicine is supposed to do.

The difference is not that one system acts and the other waits. It is that they are watching for different signals, and their red flags reflect different clinical frameworks for identifying when action is required.

THE GRAY ZONE — WHERE MOST PATIENTS ACTUALLY LIVE

Here is the honest truth about who reads books like this one: most of you are not in an emergency. You are not in crisis. Your laboratory values are not dramatically abnormal, and no one has told you that you are in immediate danger. What you have been told — often repeatedly, over a period of years — is that everything looks fine. And yet it does not feel fine.

That experience — the persistent gap between reassuring numbers and a body that is clearly under some kind of strain — is not a failure of Western Medicine to care about you. It is a structural feature of a system calibrated to detect collapse. The gray zone, where values are borderline or technically within range while symptoms persist, is not the zone Western Medicine was built to act in. "That shouldn't cause symptoms" and "Let's just watch it" are not dismissals. They are honest expressions of a system that has reached the edge of what its red flag criteria can identify.

The gray zone is not the absence of a problem. It is the presence of a problem that has not yet crossed the threshold the system was designed to recognize.

Chinese Medicine was built for the gray zone. This is not a criticism of Western Medicine — it is an acknowledgment of complementary design. Where Western Medicine identifies collapse, Chinese Medicine identifies the strain that precedes it. Functional red flags — persistent fatigue that does not resolve with rest, declining stress tolerance, poor recovery after exertion, increasing sensitivity to foods or environments, sleep that no longer restores — these changes often precede laboratory abnormalities by months or years. They are the body signaling that its compensatory capacity is being drawn down, before the compensation fails.

The patients who arrive in the most significant functional distress are rarely the ones whose labs are dramatically abnormal. They are the ones whose labs have been unremarkable for years while the body worked progressively harder to maintain those numbers. By the time a value crosses a threshold, the story has been unfolding for a while. The gray zone is where that story was being written.

Functional Red Flags — What to Notice

These are not emergency signals. They are early warning signals — the body indicating that its adaptive capacity is under increasing demand. Each one, in isolation, may be explainable. As a cluster, or as a persistent pattern over time, they deserve clinical attention:

Fatigue that does not improve with adequate rest

Declining tolerance for stress that was previously manageable

Slower recovery after illness, exertion, or emotional strain

Increasing sensitivity to foods, chemicals, or environmental triggers

Sleep that does not restore — waking unrefreshed despite sufficient hours

Symptoms that consistently worsen at specific times of day

A progressive narrowing of what the body can handle without consequence

TIMING AND THE GRAY ZONE

Timing matters in the gray zone more than anywhere else in clinical assessment. A blood draw taken during a quiet phase of the body's daily cycle does not capture peak dysfunction. A symptom that worsens consistently between 3 and 5 PM, or that reliably surfaces between 11 PM and 3 AM, is not random. It is the body's Organ Time cycle expressing a system under strain at its most active and therefore most vulnerable hour.

The clinical significance of symptom timing is something I assess in every patient encounter. A condition that worsens in the afternoon tells a different story than one present upon waking, even when laboratory values are identical. A patient who wakes consistently between 11 PM and 3 AM with racing thoughts, heat sensations, anxiety, or an urge to urinate is not describing a random sleep disturbance. They are describing Kidney and San Jiao activity at its most expressive hour.

The Kidney governs bone, bone marrow, and by extension the brain — which Chinese Medicine understands as the "sea of marrow." The San Jiao governs the water pathways of the body, including the fluid dynamics of the meninges and the cerebrospinal environment. Together, the 11 PM–3 AM window represents the body's deepest overnight regulatory work: fluid distribution through the nervous system, the fear and stress response mediated by cortisol and the adrenal axis, and the Kidney's role as the system that bears the physiological cost of sustained anxiety and chronic stress. A patient waking in this window with a racing mind, a sense of dread, or physical restlessness is often describing a Kidney system that is carrying more than it can process quietly during the hours specifically designated for that work. The morning cortisol draw will not show this at its peak. The symptom pattern does.

Fear is the Kidney's emotion in Chinese Medicine — and cortisol is its hormonal expression. In clinical practice, I often describe cortisol to patients as liquid fear: the body's chemical translation of perceived threat into physiological readiness. A patient who has been living in sustained anxiety, chronic insecurity, or prolonged stress is a patient whose Kidney system is carrying that emotional load as biochemistry — elevated cortisol, suppressed DHEA and testosterone, disrupted overnight regulation. The blood panel reflects what the body has been living. Chapter 6 maps this relationship across all seven emotions and their hormonal signatures in full.

This is why the questions patients bring to clinical encounters matter as much as the reports they carry. "What were your results?" is one question. "When do you feel worst, and what does that feel like?" is a different question — and in the gray zone, it is often the more informative one.

DISCERNMENT AS A CLINICAL SKILL

Red flags are best understood as signals that guide response, not alarms that provoke fear. Their purpose is to help determine what kind of care is needed, how urgently it is required, and which tools are appropriate at that moment. Western Medicine is designed to recognize immediate danger, structural failure, and conditions that require rapid stabilization. Chinese Medicine is designed to recognize strain, loss of coordination, and patterns that indicate the body is struggling to adapt long before collapse occurs.

These are not opposing systems. They are sequential ones. The patient with advanced kidney disease may require transplantation protocols — and may also benefit from intensive support for circulation, fluid management, and recovery capacity alongside that intervention. The patient in the gray zone may not need emergency medicine — and may benefit enormously from the kind of attentive, pattern-based clinical observation that catches what the reference ranges cannot.

Discernment, in this sense, is not about choosing sides between medical traditions. It is about recognizing where the body is on the continuum of stress, adaptation, and recovery — and responding with the level of intervention that supports health rather than undermines it. Sometimes that is a transfusion. Sometimes it is a different question asked at the right time.

Knowing which one is the work.

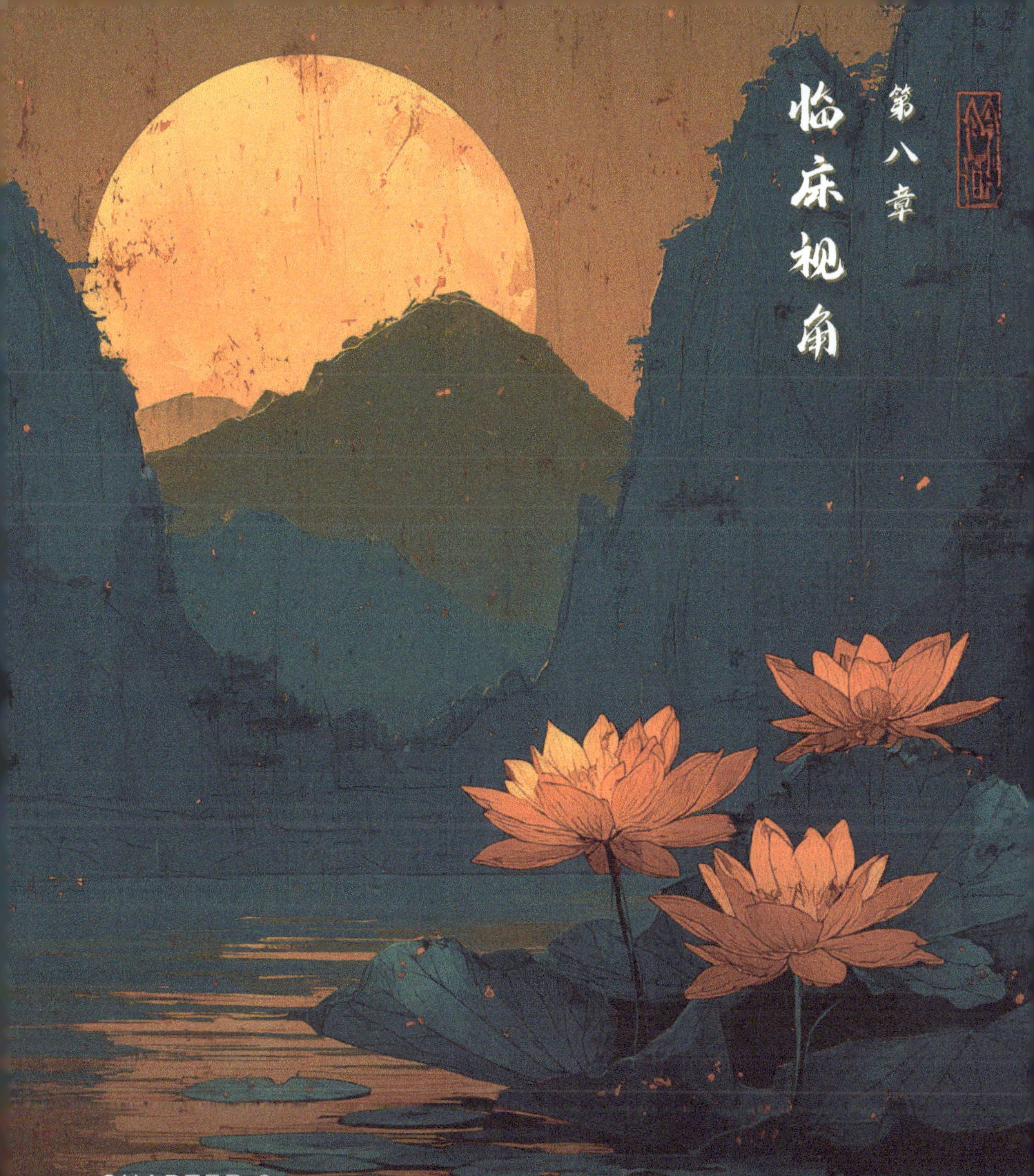

CHAPTER 8

Clinical Orientation

HOW EACH PHYSICIAN READS — AND WHY

Clinical Orientation

HOW EACH PHYSICIAN READS — AND WHY

By this point in the book, you have been introduced to a different way of understanding blood tests, symptoms, timing, and physiological strain. What may still feel unresolved is not the data itself — it is the clinical encounter. It is the moment when you hand a physician your results, or wait while they review them on a screen, and try to read from their response whether what you are experiencing is being taken seriously.

This chapter is about that moment.

When a clinician looks at your laboratory results, they are not simply reading numbers. They are operating from years of professional formation that shape what they notice first, what they consider urgent, what they feel clinically responsible for addressing, and what they are trained to set aside. These habits are not personal. They are not a reflection of how much they care about you as a patient. They are professional — which means they are systematic, consistent, and largely invisible to the person sitting on the other side of the desk.

This chapter is not about correcting physicians. I have trained in both systems and have deep respect for what each demands. It is about helping you understand how they are trained to think, so that clinical conversations become informative rather than emotionally charged — and so that a reassuring response and a concerned one can both be received as the clinical signals they actually are.

HOW WESTERN MEDICAL TRAINING SHAPES CLINICAL PERCEPTION

Medical training is not neutral observation. It is conditioning — deliberate, systematic, and designed to produce a specific kind of clinical reflexes. From the earliest stages of professional formation, Western-trained clinicians are taught to sort information quickly. The sorting process determines what requires immediate action, what requires monitoring, and what does not require intervention at all. Over time, and with repetition across thousands of patient encounters, this sorting becomes automatic. It happens before conscious deliberation.

The environments that shape Western clinical training are built around acute danger: emergency departments, hospital wards, intensive care units. The primary lesson of those environments is that failure to recognize danger has immediate and irreversible consequences. A missed sepsis. A delayed stroke. An unrecognized acute abdomen. These are the cases that become teaching moments precisely because of what happened when they were misread. The physician in training learns — at a very deep level — that the most important thing to determine, and to determine quickly, is whether something dangerous is happening right now.

This produces a clinical reflex that is genuinely lifesaving in the right context. It also produces a reflex that, in the wrong context, can feel to a patient like their experience is being dismissed.

When a Western-trained physician offers reassurance, they are communicating something precise: there is no immediate threat to life, organ integrity, or structural function. That is not the same as saying nothing is happening.

The distinction matters enormously. To a patient experiencing persistent fatigue, hormonal disruption, cognitive fog, or inflammatory pain, reassurance can feel invalidating — as though the physician did not believe them, or did not care. In most cases, neither is true. What is true is that within the Western clinical framework, nothing has crossed the threshold that obligates action. The physician is not saying your experience is imaginary. They are saying it has not yet met the criteria their system uses to justify intervention.

When red flags are present — rapidly rising kidney markers, severely abnormal electrolytes, hemoglobin below critical thresholds, inflammatory markers consistent with acute infection — urgency appears immediately in tone, behavior, and intervention. The same physician who offered measured reassurance at a previous visit will be direct and decisive when the data calls for it. That shift is not inconsistency. It is the system working as designed.

Understanding this allows patients to interpret clinical responses as information about how their condition is being categorized — not as a personal verdict on whether their experience is real.

HOW CHINESE MEDICINE TRAINING SHAPES CLINICAL PERCEPTION

Chinese Medicine follows a different training pathway, shaped by different clinical priorities and a different set of founding questions. Where Western clinical training asks above all else whether something dangerous is happening right now, Chinese Medicine training asks a different first question:

> *How hard is the body working*
> *to maintain regulation?*

This is not a lesser question. It is a differently oriented one. A value within reference range may still carry significant clinical meaning if it requires excessive effort to sustain. Symptoms are not treated as secondary to laboratory data but as part of the same diagnostic field — equal in weight, sometimes superior in specificity. Timing, rhythm, and recovery capacity are weighted heavily in the clinical assessment. The Four Examinations — looking, listening, asking, and touching — are not supplementary to laboratory findings. They are the primary clinical instrument, with laboratory values functioning as confirmation and clarification.

This training produces a clinical orientation that is genuinely distinct from the Western one — not better, not worse, but calibrated to notice different signals first. A Chinese Medicine physician looking at the same CBC, metabolic panel, and lipid results as a Western physician is asking different questions of the same data. One is asking whether the organ has failed. The other is asking how efficiently the organ is functioning and what it is costing the body to maintain that function.

Sitting with both sets of clinical reflexes simultaneously is illuminating in a way that is difficult to fully convey. The same patient, the same report, the same numbers. Two legitimate clinical frameworks, each catching something the other is not calibrated to see. The gap between them is not a failure of either system. It is a description of what integration actually makes possible.

WHY DIFFERENT CLINICIANS RESPOND DIFFERENTLY TO THE SAME DATA

Patients frequently experience confusion when two clinicians respond very differently to the same laboratory results. One appears unconcerned. Another takes the same values seriously. One recommends watchful waiting. Another recommends immediate intervention. The temptation is to conclude that one of them is wrong, or that medicine is less certain than it presents itself to be.

Both responses may be entirely correct within their respective frameworks. A Western-trained physician who sees values within reference range and recommends observation is responding from a mandate that defines action thresholds in terms of structural danger. A Chinese Medicine physician who sees the same values and recommends intervention is responding from a mandate that defines action thresholds in terms of functional strain and compensatory effort. Neither is making an error. They are answering different questions.

Reading Clinical Responses as Signals

Heightened urgency — *a shift in tone, immediate referral, or rapid intervention — signals that the clinician has identified something in the data that crosses their system's threshold for dangerous or rapidly progressing.*

Measured reassurance *signals that within that clinician's framework, the condition does not currently meet criteria for intervention. This is not the same as nothing being present.*

Watchful waiting *signals uncertainty combined with low immediate risk — the clinician cannot yet* *determine which direction the pattern is heading and is gathering more information before acting.*

These are not evaluations of your experience. They are professional sortings of your data. Receiving them as such removes a considerable amount of the emotional charge from clinical encounters.

Bedside manner, in this context, is often an expression of clinical orientation rather than personal disposition. A physician who appears calm and unworried when you feel anything but is not necessarily indifferent. They may be operating from a framework in which your condition, while uncomfortable for you, does not currently represent the kind of danger that their training obliges them to act on. That is useful information. It tells you where your condition sits within their clinical map, which in turn tells you something about what kind of additional inquiry might be appropriate.

The patient who understands this is considerably better equipped to navigate the healthcare system than the one who interprets every reassurance as dismissal and every expression of concern as catastrophe. Both responses — from the clinician and from the patient — are more useful when they are understood as clinical signals rather than personal ones.

USING THIS UNDERSTANDING IN CLINICAL CONVERSATIONS

The most practical application of what this chapter offers is a shift in how you listen during clinical encounters. Rather than listening for whether the physician validates your experience — which places the entire weight of the interaction on an emotional outcome — listen for what their response is telling you about how your condition is being categorized.

Is this being treated as an emergency? Then something in the data has crossed a threshold that requires action. Follow that lead.

Is this being met with reassurance and observation? Then within that framework, you are not in immediate danger. That is genuinely good information. It also leaves open the question of whether you are in the gray zone — the compensating, straining, functional-strain territory that Chapter 7 described — and whether a different clinical lens might add something to that picture.

The questions that tend to produce the most useful clinical conversations are the ones that invite the physician into a different level of the inquiry. Not "Why don't you believe me?" but "I understand the results are within range — is there a pattern in these values over time that would be worth tracking?" Not "Is something wrong?" but "Is there anything here that could explain why I feel consistently worse at a particular time of day?"

These are not confrontational questions. They are precise ones. And precision, in a clinical encounter, tends to produce more useful answers than frustration — even when the frustration is entirely justified.

ORIENTATION AS A CLINICAL TOOL

Understanding how physicians are trained to read data does not require you to agree with every clinical decision you encounter. It requires only that you receive those decisions as products of a framework rather than as personal responses to you as a patient. That shift — from personal to professional, from emotional to informational — changes what is possible in the clinical conversation.

It allows care to be escalated when the situation calls for it, without the patient needing to fight for that escalation through emotional channels. It allows reassurance to land as the genuinely useful information it often is, rather than as a door closing. And it allows the patient who is in the gray zone — whose experience exceeds what a single clinical framework can fully account for — to ask the kinds of questions that open the door to a more complete picture.

Chapter 9 moves directly into that picture. It will address how reference ranges are constructed, what they can and cannot tell you, and how both Western Medicine and Chinese Medicine interpret the same numerical data through different lenses. With the orientation this chapter provides, that information can be received as a tool rather than a verdict.

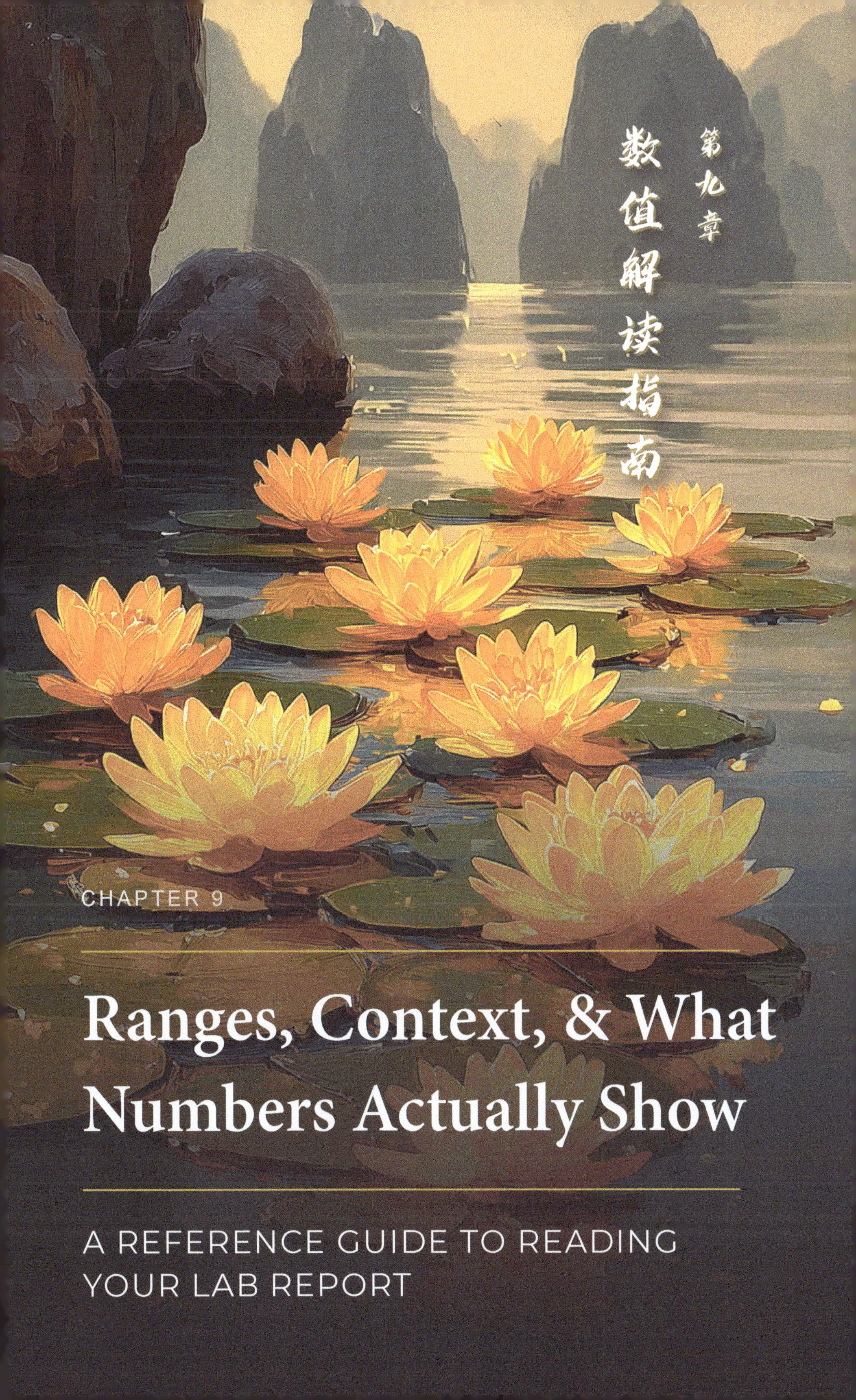

第九章

数值解读指南

CHAPTER 9

Ranges, Context, & What Numbers Actually Show

A REFERENCE GUIDE TO READING YOUR LAB REPORT

Ranges, Context, & What Numbers Actually Show

A REFERENCE GUIDE TO READING YOUR LAB REPORT

Most people encounter their laboratory results alone. A report appears in a patient portal or arrives by email. Numbers are listed in columns. Some are highlighted, others are not. A reference range is printed beside each value, but rarely explained. There is no immediate context for what is being measured, why it matters, or how seriously to take it.

That moment — alone with a report full of numbers you were not taught to read — is where confusion most often begins. And confusion, in the absence of context, tends to move in one of two directions: either toward dismissal ("everything looks fine, nothing to worry about") or toward alarm ("something is flagged, something must be wrong"). Neither response is particularly useful when the actual clinical picture is more nuanced than a flag or the absence of one.

This chapter is designed to be used as a reference. You do not need to read it straight through. Return to it when a value on your report feels unfamiliar, when a number has been flagged and you want to understand what that flag actually means, or when you want to compare what Western Medicine and Chinese Medicine observe in the same marker. Its purpose is orientation — replacing guesswork with understanding, so that when you sit with a physician to discuss your results, you are a participant in the conversation rather than an audience for it.

> *Laboratory ranges describe boundaries, not health. They show where regulation holds — not how it feels to maintain it.*

WHAT A LAB REPORT ACTUALLY CONTAINS

Before interpreting any value, it helps to understand what the report is and is not showing you. A standard laboratory report contains five elements, and each one means something specific.

The Five Elements of A Lab Report

Test Name — Identifies what is being measured. The name alone does not indicate importance or urgency — only category.

Result — The measured value at the time of collection. This reflects a single moment, not a trend. The same value drawn at a different hour may look different.

Reference Range — A statistical interval based on population data. It indicates where most values fall, not what is optimal for an individual. Ranges vary between laboratories.

Flag or Indicator — A visual marker showing that a value falls outside the laboratory's predefined range. A flag signals that attention may be warranted — not a diagnosis or emergency on its own.

Units of Measurement — Units describe scale, not severity. A value in nanograms per milliliter is not more alarming than one in grams per deciliter simply because the number appears smaller.

UNITS OF MEASUREMENT — A QUICK REFERENCE

Laboratory reports use standardized units that reflect measurement precision, not clinical severity. Smaller numbers with smaller units do not indicate less concern, and larger numbers with larger units do not indicate more. Here is a plain-language guide to the units you will most commonly encounter.

Common Lab Units — What They Mean in Plain Language

cells/mm³ (cmm) — Cells per cubic millimeter — how many cells are present in a very small volume of blood

fL (femtoliter) — One quadrillionth of a liter — used to measure the size of individual red blood cells (MCV)

g/dL — Grams per deciliter — weight of a substance per tenth of a liter of blood; used for hemoglobin and albumin

IU/L — International units per liter — a standardized unit for enzyme activity; used for liver enzymes and thyroid markers

mEq/L — Milliequivalents per liter — measures the chemical activity of electrolytes like sodium and potassium

mg/dL — Milligrams per deciliter — weight per tenth of a liter; used for glucose, cholesterol, creatinine, and bilirubin

mmol/L — Millimoles per liter- a molecular measure used for electrolytes in many non-US laboratory systems

ng/mL — Nanograms per milliliter — an extremely small weight measure; used for hormones including testosterone and Hormone D3

pg/mL — Picograms per milliliter — smaller still; used for estradiol, free T3, and other highly sensitive hormone measures

U/L — Units per liter — enzyme activity measure; used for ALT, AST, and alkaline phosphatase

HOW EACH SYSTEM READS THE SAME REPORT

Western Medicine and Chinese Medicine are not reading different reports. They are asking different questions of the same one.

From a Western Medicine perspective, the first question is whether any value indicates immediate risk, structural failure, or disease requiring intervention. If the answer is no, the report is typically categorized as stable. This is appropriate and clinically sound within that framework. It identifies what the reference ranges were designed to identify.

From a Chinese Medicine perspective, attention moves toward patterns: values clustering near the edges of their ranges, relationships between markers across panels, the timing of collection relative to the body's daily physiological cycle, and how the numbers correspond with what the patient is experiencing. A value at the low end of its reference range is not the same clinical picture as a value in the middle of its range, even when both are technically "normal." One may reflect regulation maintained with effort. The other may reflect regulation maintained with ease. That distinction does not appear in the flag column.

Functional Definitions- How to Read the Range

Within range — Regulation is being maintained at the time of measurement. This does not describe how much effort that maintenance requires.

High-normal / Low-normal — Balance is being maintained at the edge of the system's comfortable operating range. Worth noting as a trend marker.

Borderline — An early signal of strain or adaptation. The body is compensating. Not yet flagged, but worth clinical attention — particularly if accompanied by symptoms.

Flagged — The value has crossed the laboratory's statistical threshold. Closer observation or correlation is warranted. Does not by itself constitute a diagnosis.

Trending — A value moving consistently in one direction across multiple draws — even while remaining within range — often carries more clinical significance than a single flagged result.

PANEL REFERENCE GUIDE

The tables that follow present the most commonly ordered laboratory panels with reference ranges, Western Medicine functional interpretation, and Chinese Medicine functional interpretation for each marker. These ranges are illustrative — they reflect typical adult values and will vary between laboratories and individual patient contexts. Use them to orient yourself, not to reach conclusions independently.

A note before reading: the Chinese Medicine interpretations in these tables draw on thirty years of clinical practice integrating both frameworks. They are not replacements for the Western values — they are additions to them, describing what the same number may reflect from a different clinical vantage point.

COMPLETE BLOOD COUNT - CBC

Marker Reference Guide — Western Medicine & Chinese Medicine Functional Views

> What it observes: Blood production, oxygen transport, immune engagement, and containment. The CBC reflects the quantity and functional capacity of the body's three primary blood cell populations.

Marker / Reference Range	Western Medicine View	Chinese Medicine View
Red Blood Cells (RBC) *Women: ~4.2–5.4 million cells/μL* *Men: ~4.7–6.1 million cells/μL*	Reflects the number of circulating red blood cells available for oxygen transport. Low counts suggest reduced delivery capacity.	Relates to the sufficiency of Blood (血, Xuè). Low-normal trends may suggest Blood is being maintained with effort rather than abundance — even when hemoglobin appears adequate.

Marker / Reference Range	Western Medicine View	Chinese Medicine View
Hemoglobin *Women: ~12.0–15.5 g/dL* *Men: ~13.5–17.5 g/dL*	Reflects oxygen-carrying capacity. The primary marker for anemia classification.	Associated with nourishment and vitality of Blood. Values near the lower end of the range may correspond to fatigue, poor concentration, or palpitations even when technically normal.
Hematocrit *Women: ~36–48%* *Men: ~41–53%*	Percentage of blood volume made up of red blood cells. Rises and falls with hemoglobin.	May reflect Blood concentration or fluid balance. Low-normal values alongside adequate hemoglobin may indicate fluid distribution issues rather than true anemia.
White Blood Cells (WBC) *~4.0–11.0 ×10⁹/L*	Reflects immune engagement and inflammatory signaling. Elevated counts suggest active response; suppressed counts may indicate immune compromise or bone marrow strain.	Represents Wei Qi (卫气, Wèi Qì) — Defensive Qi activity. Chronic elevation may reflect sustained immune demand; chronic suppression may reflect depletion of defensive capacity rather than simple immune insufficiency.
Platelets *~150–450 ×10⁹/L*	Supports clotting and vascular integrity. Low counts suggest bleeding risk; elevated counts may reflect inflammatory or reactive production.	Relates to Blood containment and stability. High-normal values may reflect low-grade inflammation or Qi Stagnation. Low-normal values may reflect Blood or Fluid depletion reducing recovery capacity.

THYROID PROFILE

Marker Reference Guide — Western Medicine & Chinese Medicine Functional Views

What it observes: Metabolic signaling and energy regulation. Thyroid markers reflect not only hormone production but the efficiency of conversion and delivery to target tissues — a sequence that can be disrupted without producing flagged values.

Marker / Reference Range	Western Medicine View	Chinese Medicine View
TSH (Thyroid-Stimulating Hormone) *~0.4–4.0 mIU/L*	Reflects how much signaling the pituitary is sending to maintain thyroid hormone levels. Elevated TSH suggests the thyroid is being asked to work harder. Suppressed TSH suggests overproduction or exogenous hormone.	Represents regulatory effort rather than output. A high-normal TSH in a symptomatic patient may reflect compensation — the system working harder to maintain function — before values cross diagnostic thresholds.
Free T4 (Thyroxine) *~0.8–1.8 ng/dL*	Represents circulating thyroid hormone in its reserve form. Must be converted to Free T3 to become metabolically active.	Relates to metabolic potential and reserve. Adequate Free T4 with low-normal Free T3 suggests conversion impairment — the production is present but the delivery is not completing.
Free T3 (Triiodothyronine) *~2.3–4.2 pg/mL*	Represents active thyroid hormone available to tissues. Drives metabolism, temperature regulation, and cognitive speed.	Reflects expression and distribution of metabolic activity. Low-normal Free T3 with normal TSH and T4 is a common pattern in patients with cold sensitivity, fatigue, and cognitive slowing — a conversion problem, not a production problem.

HORMONE PANEL

What it observes: Hormonal signaling, timing, and coordination between systems. Hormone values describe whether signals are being produced, but also how much effort is required to maintain regulation. Because hormones function rhythmically, single measurements capture a moment rather than a pattern.

Marker / Reference Range	Western Medicine View	Chinese Medicine View
Cortisol (Morning) *~5–25 μg/dL* *(drawn 8–9 AM)*	Reflects stress response and energy mobilization. The morning cortisol awakening response should represent the day's peak. A low morning value may reflect blunted awakening response; an elevated evening value (not captured by standard draw) may reflect dysregulated rhythm.	Represents adaptive Yang activity. Rhythm and timing carry more clinical information than a single value. A within-range morning cortisol does not confirm a healthy cortisol curve — it confirms the value at one point on that curve.
Estradiol (Estrogen) *Women: Follicular: ~30–120 pg/mL* *Mid-cycle: ~130–370 pg/mL* *Luteal: ~70–250 pg/mL* *Postmenopausal: <30 pg/mL* *Men: ~10–40 pg/mL*	Reflects reproductive and tissue signaling. Must be interpreted in context of menstrual cycle day — a value appropriate for one phase may be insufficient for another.	Associated with Yin nourishment and Blood movement. Low-normal estradiol with intact cycle may reflect Blood Deficiency or Liver constraint impairing smooth hormonal distribution.
Progesterone (Luteal Phase) *Women: Follicular: <1 ng/mL* *Luteal: ~5–20 ng/mL* *Postmenopausal: <1 ng/mL* *Men: <1 ng/mL*	Reflects post-ovulatory hormonal support. Adequate luteal progesterone is required for sleep quality, mood stability, and cycle regulation.	Associated with Yin containment and stability. Low progesterone despite ovulation may reflect insufficient Yin or Kidney reserve to sustain the luteal phase.

Marker / Reference Range	Western Medicine View	Chinese Medicine View
Testosterone *Women: ~15–70 ng/dL* *Men: ~300–1,000 ng/dL*	Reflects anabolic signaling and vitality. Follows a diurnal pattern — values are highest in the early morning and decline 25–50% by late afternoon. Time of draw matters significantly for borderline values.	Associated with Yang expression and vitality. Low-normal testosterone in a patient with fatigue, low motivation, and cold sensitivity may reflect Kidney Yang depletion rather than primary gonadal insufficiency.
Hormone D3 (Cholecalciferol) *~30–80 ng/mL (optimal)* *<20 ng/mL (deficient)*	Reflects availability of the active steroid hormone converted from UV-synthesized precursors via the liver and kidneys. Governs calcium metabolism, immune regulation, and inflammatory signaling.	Understood through the biliary bone matrix — the Liver and Gallbladder conversion pathway. Deficiency despite adequate sun exposure often reflects impaired hepatic or biliary conversion rather than insufficient precursor.

LIVER FUNCTION PANEL

What it observes: Metabolic workload, transformation, and clearance. The liver function panel reflects how efficiently the body processes nutrients, hormones, medications, and waste products. A value within range may still reflect strain if workload is elevated or clearance is inefficient.

Marker / Reference Range	Western Medicine View	Chinese Medicine View
AST (Aspartate Aminotransferase) *~10–40 U/L*	Reflects liver cell stress or metabolic demand. Elevated values prompt evaluation for hepatitis, medication toxicity, or muscle injury (AST is also present in cardiac and skeletal muscle).	May reflect strain in Liver coursing and adaptation. Persistent high-normal AST in the absence of structural cause suggests the Liver is processing at capacity.
ALT (Alanine Aminotransferase) *~7–56 U/L*	More specific to liver cell stress than AST. The primary marker for hepatic workload and cellular injury.	Associated with constrained Liver Qi movement or internal heat. Mild, persistent high-normal ALT often corresponds to chronic emotional strain, hormonal burden, or impaired fat metabolism.
Bilirubin (Total) *~0.1–1.2 mg/dL*	Reflects red blood cell breakdown and liver processing capacity. Elevated values may indicate hemolysis, liver dysfunction, or biliary obstruction.	Understood through the Liver's regulation of smooth Blood movement. Elevated bilirubin in Chinese Medicine may reflect Damp-Heat obstruction or digestive strain affecting bile flow.
Albumin *~3.5–5.0 g/dL*	A protein produced by the liver that maintains fluid balance and transports substances in the blood. Low albumin indicates reduced liver synthetic capacity.	Relates to the Spleen's role in transformation and the Liver's role in distribution. Low albumin alongside fatigue and digestive weakness may reflect Spleen Qi deficiency affecting protein metabolism.

METABOLIC PANEL

What it observes: The stability of the body's internal environment. The metabolic panel reflects how the body regulates fluids, electrolytes, energy availability, and waste clearance. A value within range may still reflect increased effort if balance is sustained through compensation.

Marker / Reference Range	Western Medicine View	Chinese Medicine View
Glucose (Fasting) *~70–99 mg/dL*	Reflects circulating fuel availability at baseline. Used to screen for diabetes and hypoglycemia. Does not capture afternoon or post-prandial glucose regulation.	Reflects energy regulation capacity and Liver-Spleen functional relationship. Fasting glucose in range alongside afternoon energy instability suggests Spleen Qi strain — a pattern the morning draw does not capture.
Sodium *~135–145 mmol/L*	Primary electrolyte governing fluid balance and nerve conduction. Significant deviation indicates fluid dysregulation requiring prompt attention.	Reflects the body's internal fluid distribution. Low-normal sodium may indicate chronic Spleen Qi deficiency affecting fluid transformation and transportation.
Potassium *~3.5–5.0 mmol/L*	Governs cardiac rhythm and muscle contraction. Even borderline low values warrant clinical attention in patients with cardiac history.	Borderline potassium alongside fatigue, palpitations, or reduced stress tolerance may reflect Yin deficiency — insufficient cellular moisture and containment.

Marker / Reference Range	Western Medicine View	Chinese Medicine View
Creatinine *Women: ~0.5–1.1 mg/dL* *Men: ~0.7–1.3 mg/dL*	A waste product filtered by the kidneys. Rising creatinine indicates reduced filtration capacity. Trends within range matter as much as absolute values.	Does not directly reflect Kidney Jing (精, Jīng) — the deep constitutional reserve. A slowly rising creatinine within range, alongside fatigue and declining endurance, may signal Kidney reserve under increasing demand.
BUN (Blood Urea Nitrogen) *~7–20 mg/dL*	Reflects protein metabolism and kidney filtration efficiency. Elevated BUN with elevated creatinine suggests reduced kidney function.	Observed in relation to Kidney function and fluid metabolism. Elevated BUN in the context of dehydration or high protein intake should be distinguished from elevated BUN reflecting genuine filtration decline.

Reference ranges reflect typical adult values and vary between laboratories. Use these values to orient clinical interpretation — not to reach independent conclusions. Always bring findings to a qualified healthcare professional.

HOW TO USE THIS CHAPTER

Return to these tables when a value on your report raises a question. Use the Western Medicine column to understand what the marker is measuring and what a flagged or borderline result typically prompts clinically. Use the Chinese Medicine column to understand what the same value may reflect from a functional perspective — what it says about how the body is managing the demands being placed on it, and at what cost.

Do not read isolated numbers. Do not assign meaning to a single flag. Do not assume that the absence of disease means the absence of strain. Use the ranges to orient yourself, not to reach conclusions.

And always — always — bring your questions to a qualified healthcare professional who can place these values in the context of your full clinical picture. This chapter improves the quality of that conversation. It does not replace it.

REGIONAL MEDICAL LABORATORY
1200 Health Sciences Blvd · Orlando, FL 32827 · (407) 555-0182

February 14, 2026
Collected: 07:45 AM
• ALL RESULTS WITHIN RANGE

PATIENT NAME	DOB / SEX	ORDERING PROVIDER	SPECIMEN TYPE
Joanne Smith	06/06/1981 · F	J. Smith, M.D.	Whole Blood · Routine

COLLECTION DATE	COLLECTION TIME	SPECIMEN #	FASTING STATUS
02/14/2026	07:45 AM	4567332	Yes · 12 hrs

Morning fasting draw

✓ WITHIN NORMAL RANGE

- All 17 values within reference range. No flags present. Results reflect morning fasting baseline.

COMPLETE BLOOD COUNT (CBC) — with Differential

TEST	RESULT	UNITS	REFERENCE RANGE	RANGE POSITION
White Blood Cell WBC	**6.2**	K/µL	4.0 - 11.0	
Red Blood Cell RBC	**4.8**	M/µL	4.2 - 5.4	
Hemoglobin HGB	**13.4**	g/dL	12.0 - 16.0	
Hematocrit HCT	**40.1**	%	36.0 - 46.0	
Mean Cell Volume MCV	**88**	fL	80 - 100	
Platelet Count PLT	**242**	K/µL	150 - 400	

COMPREHENSIVE METABOLIC PANEL (CMP)

TEST	RESULT	UNITS	REFERENCE RANGE	RANGE POSITION
Glucose, Fasting	**88**	mg/dL	70 - 99	
Creatinine	**0.82**	mg/dL	0.60 - 1.10	
ALT (Alanine Aminotransferase)	**24**	U/L	7 - 56	
Sodium	**139**	mmol/L	135 - 145	
Potassium	**4.1**	mmol/L	3.5 - 5.0	

THYROID & HORMONES

TEST	RESULT	UNITS	REFERENCE RANGE	RANGE POSITION
TSH (Thyroid Stimulating Hormone)	**2.1**	mIU/L	0.40 - 4.00	
Free T4 (Thyroxine)	**1.2**	ng/dL	0.80 - 1.80	
Free T3 (Triiodothyronine)	**3.1**	pg/mL	2.30 - 4.20	
Cortisol (Morning)	**18.4**	µg/dL	6.0 - 23.0	
Hormone D3 (25-Hydroxyvitamin D)	**44**	ng/mL	30 - 100	
C-Reactive Protein (hs-CRP)	**0.8**	mg/L	< 3.0	

This report is for educational orientation purposes. Values reflect a morning fasting collection. Reference ranges are population-based statistical intervals and do not define individual health or optimal function. Always review results with a qualified clinician.

Report #RML-2026-021401
Verified 02/14/2026 · 09:18 AM

REGIONAL MEDICAL LABORATORY
1200 Health Sciences Blvd · Orlando, FL 32827 · (407) 555-0182

March 3, 2026
Collected: 08:20 AM
⚠ REVIEW REQUIRED · 6 FLAGS

PATIENT NAME	DOB / SEX	ORDERING PROVIDER	SPECIMEN TYPE
Marcus Johnson	11/14/1974 · M	A. Rivera, M.D.	Whole Blood · Routine

COLLECTION DATE	COLLECTION TIME	SPECIMEN #	FASTING STATUS
03/03/2026	08:20 AM	4571890	Yes · 10 hrs

⚠ 6 values outside reference range

⚠ VALUES OUTSIDE REFERENCE RANGE

- 6 of 17 values flagged. A flag indicates statistical difference — not automatic disease. Review with your clinician.

COMPLETE BLOOD COUNT (CBC) — with Differential

TEST	RESULT	UNITS	REFERENCE RANGE	RANGE POSITION
White Blood Cell WBC	7.4	K/µL	4.0 - 11.0	
Red Blood Cell RBC	4.9	M/µL	4.5 - 5.9	
Hemoglobin HGB	14.8	g/dL	13.5 - 17.5	
Hematocrit HCT	44.2	%	41.0 - 53.0	
Mean Cell Volume MCV	86	fL	80 - 100	
Platelet Count PLT	188	K/µL	150 - 400	

COMPREHENSIVE METABOLIC PANEL (CMP)

TEST	RESULT	UNITS	REFERENCE RANGE	RANGE POSITION
Glucose, Fasting	108 H	mg/dL	70 - 99	
Creatinine	1.02	mg/dL	0.74 - 1.35	
ALT (Alanine Aminotransferase)	72 H	U/L	7 - 56	
Sodium	141	mmol/L	135 - 145	
Potassium	4.3	mmol/L	3.5 - 5.0	

THYROID & HORMONES

TEST	RESULT	UNITS	REFERENCE RANGE	RANGE POSITION
TSH (Thyroid Stimulating Hormone)	5.2 H	mIU/L	0.40 - 4.00	
Free T4 (Thyroxine)	0.9	ng/dL	0.80 - 1.80	
Free T3 (Triiodothyronine)	2.8	pg/mL	2.30 - 4.20	
Cortisol (Morning)	28.6 H	µg/dL	6.0 - 23.0	
Hormone D3 (25-Hydroxyvitamin D)	16 L	ng/mL	30 - 100	
C-Reactive Protein (hs-CRP)	2.6	mg/L	< 3.0	

Flagged values fall outside population-based reference ranges. A flag indicates statistical difference — not automatic disease or emergency. Results should always be interpreted alongside symptoms, timing of collection, and full clinical context by a qualified provider.

Report #RML-2026-030301
Verified 03/03/2026 · 10:06 AM

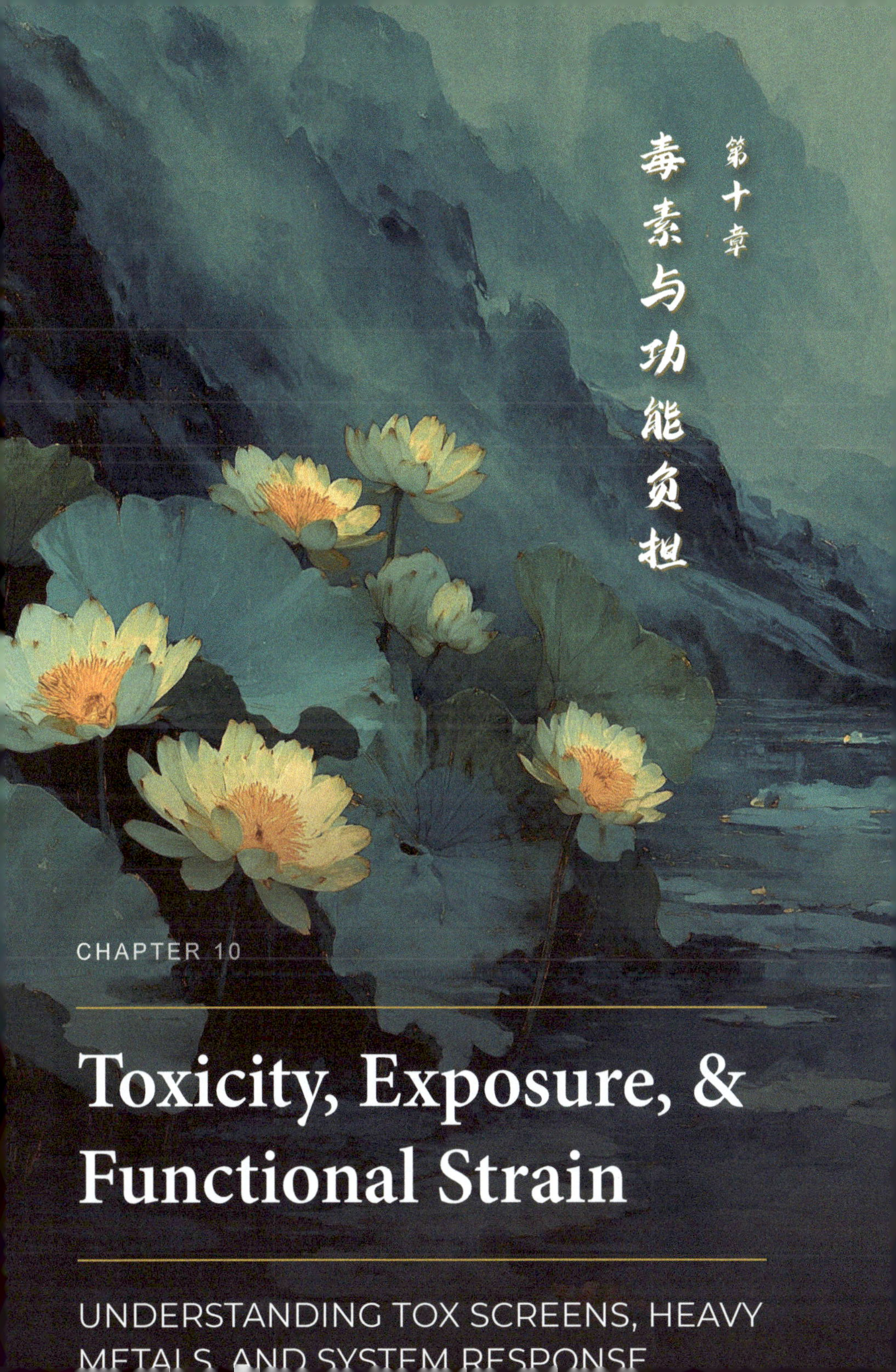

第十章

毒素与功能负担

CHAPTER 10

Toxicity, Exposure, & Functional Strain

UNDERSTANDING TOX SCREENS, HEAVY METALS, AND SYSTEM RESPONSE

Toxicity, Exposure, & Functional Strain

UNDERSTANDING TOX SCREENS, HEAVY METALS, AND SYSTEM RESPONSE

Toxicology results are among the most anxiety-producing laboratory findings a patient can receive — and among the most misread. A detectable value for lead, mercury, or arsenic triggers an alarm response that the number alone rarely justifies. Conversely, results reported as "non-detectable" are sometimes treated as complete reassurance when they represent only the absence of acute, measurable accumulation — not the absence of functional burden.

Both reactions — alarm and dismissal — share the same root: interpreting a presence or absence of a substance as though it were, by itself, a clinical conclusion. It is not. Toxicology tests measure what is present and at what concentration. They do not measure what the body is doing with it, how it is responding to it, or what the cumulative functional cost of that response has been over time.

That is what this chapter addresses. Not to alarm, and

not to reassure prematurely — but to provide the clinical framework that turns a toxicology result from an abstraction into a meaningful piece of a larger picture.

> *Presence does not define outcome. Pattern and system response provide meaning.*

HOW EACH SYSTEM APPROACHES EXPOSURE

Western toxicology measures the concentration of substances in blood, urine, or tissue and compares those values against population-based reference ranges. This framework is designed to identify recent or ongoing exposure, observe accumulation patterns over time, and determine whether concentrations are approaching levels associated with known physiological harm. A detectable value indicates that a substance is present. It does not, by itself, indicate injury, disease, or prognosis. Reference ranges guide further evaluation — they do not provide conclusions on their own.

Chinese Medicine approaches exposure differently. Rather than evaluating the substance alone, it evaluates how the body is responding to it. The presence of a heavy metal or environmental toxin becomes clinically relevant not primarily because of its chemical identity, but because of the functional disruption it is generating — which system relationships it is straining, which physiological processes it is burdening, and whether the body has sufficient reserve to manage and clear the load being placed on it.

Two frameworks organize this interpretation.

六邪气 Liù Xié Qì — The Six Excesses: How Disruption Expresses

Wind (风, Fēng) — Instability, reactivity, tremor, sudden change — neurological and movement disruption

Cold (寒, Hán) — Slowing, fatigue, constriction, reduced warmth — metabolic suppression and circulatory stagnation

Heat (热, Rè) — Inflammation, agitation, restlessness — excitatory and inflammatory responses

Dampness (湿, Shī) — Heaviness, fogginess, sluggish transformation — impaired fluid metabolism and cognitive clarity

Dryness (燥, Zào) — Depletion, irritation, lack of nourishment — tissue depletion and moisture loss

Summer-Heat (暑, Shǔ) — Exhaustion with agitation or collapse — acute depletion under sustained demand

藏象 Zàng Xiàng — Organ System Relationships in Exposure

Liver (肝, Gān) — Governs movement, adaptation, and regulation — the primary detoxification and hormonal clearance system

Spleen (脾, Pí) — Governs transformation and transport — processes nutrients and manages Damp accumulation

Kidney (肾, Shèn) — Governs storage and long-term reserve — determines resilience and recovery capacity under prolonged burden

Heart (心, Xīn) — Governs circulation and mental integration (Shen) — affected when exposure disrupts neurological or emotional stability

Lung (肺, Fèi) — Governs boundary, rhythm, and sensitivity — the body's first interface with airborne and environmental exposure

A NOTE ON UNITS IN TOXICOLOGY REPORTS

Toxicology results are frequently reported in very small units that can make values appear more alarming than they are — or, conversely, so small that patients assume they are negligible. Neither assumption is clinically sound. The unit describes measurement precision, not severity.

Toxicology Units — Plain Language

μg/dL (micrograms per deciliter) — Millionths of a gram per tenth of a liter of blood — used for lead and some other metals in blood

μg/L (micrograms per liter) — Millionths of a gram per full liter — used for mercury and arsenic in blood or urine

μg/g creatinine — Adjusts urinary metal levels for urine concentration — a more stable measure than urine concentration alone

Non-detectable — Below the laboratory's detection threshold. Does not mean absent — means not measurable at this level of sensitivity

HEAVY METAL PROFILES

The following profiles present the four most commonly tested heavy metals with Western functional interpretation, Chinese Medicine functional interpretation, and the organ system relationships most commonly involved in exposure patterns. These profiles are reference material — not diagnostic criteria. Interpretation of actual exposure results should always involve a qualified clinician with access to the full clinical picture.

Lead (Pb)

Reference range: <5 μg/dL (blood) — micrograms per deciliter

Western Medicine

Lead interferes with neurological signaling, red blood cell formation, and kidney regulation. Even low-level chronic exposure can present gradually, affecting cognitive function, mood, and immune competence before laboratory values cross alert thresholds. In children, no safe level of lead exposure has been established.

Chinese Medicine

Understood as Damp-Heat obstructing smooth movement and burdening Blood regulation. The combination of Dampness and Heat produces the characteristic pattern of heaviness, cognitive fog, and inflammatory reactivity — without the acute presentation that might prompt immediate clinical concern.

六邪气 Liù Xié Qì Expression

- Dampness - heaviness, fogginess, sluggish processing

- Heat — inflammation, irritability, restlessness
- Wind — neurological reactivity, tremor, instability

藏象 Zàng Xiàng Involvement

- Liver — movement and adaptation under toxic burden
- Spleen — transformation and Damp management
- Heart — Shen disturbance when irritability and cognitive fog are prominent

Common Functional Tendencies

- Cognitive fog and difficulty concentrating
- Fatigue that does not respond normally to rest
- Head pressure or dull headache
- Irritability disproportionate to circumstances
- Digestive heaviness and sluggishness

MERCURY (Hg)

Reference range: <10 µg/L (blood) — micrograms per liter

Western Medicine

Mercury affects nervous system signaling and immune regulation. Organic forms — particularly methylmercury from fish consumption — accumulate more readily in tissue and cross the blood-brain barrier. Inorganic mercury from dental amalgam or occupational exposure follows a different distribution pattern. The form of mercury matters as much as the level.

Chinese Medicine

Associated with internal Wind, Yin strain, and Shen disturbance. Mercury's neurological affinity aligns closely with Wind patterns in Chinese Medicine — the instability, tremor, and unpredictability that characterize Wind expression. The Yin depletion component reflects mercury's tendency to generate heat and dryness in the nervous system over time.

六邪气 Liù Xié Qì Expression

- Wind — neurological instability, tremor,
- internal vibration
- Heat — agitation, restlessness, inflammatory sensitivity
- Dryness — tissue depletion, lack of
- nourishment, sensory irritability

藏象 Zàng Xiàng Involvement

- Liver — movement and detoxification
- Heart — Shen stability and mental integration

- Kidney — Yin support and long-term nourishment of the nervous system
- Common Functional Tendencies
- Tremor or a sensation of internal vibration
- Sleep disturbance — difficulty staying asleep or achieving deep rest
- Heightened sensory sensitivity — to light, sound, smell, or touch
- Emotional variability disproportionate to external circumstances
- Cognitive changes, particularly in memory and word retrieval

ARSENIC (As)

Reference range: <50 µg/L (urine) — reflects recent exposure; organic forms from seafood may elevate without toxicological significance

Western Medicine

Arsenic interferes with cellular energy production and vascular function. Inorganic arsenic — from contaminated water, soil, or occupational exposure — is the form of primary clinical concern. Organic arsenic from seafood is generally less toxic and clears rapidly. Speciation testing, which distinguishes organic from inorganic forms, is clinically important when urine arsenic is elevated.

Chinese Medicine

Associated with Damp-Heat affecting transformation and circulation. The vascular and skin manifestations of arsenic exposure align with Chinese Medicine patterns of Damp obstruction and Heat in the Blood — producing the combination of circulatory impairment, skin changes, and digestive irregularity that characterizes chronic low-level exposure.

六邪气 Liù Xié Qì Expression

- Dampness — heaviness, sluggish transformation, fluid accumulation
- Heat — inflammation, skin reactivity, circulatory agitation

藏象 Zàng Xiàng Involvement

- Spleen — transformation and Damp
- management
- Liver — movement and circulatory regulation

Common Functional Tendencies

- Digestive irregularity — nausea, cramping,
- altered bowel function
- Skin changes — hyperpigmentation, keratosis, or unusual texture changes

- Fatigue with circulatory component — heaviness in the limbs, poor peripheral warmth
- Circulatory discomfort — numbness, tingling, or vascular sensitivity

CADMIUM (Cd)

Reference range: <1 μg/L (blood) — reflects longer-term accumulation; urine cadmium reflects kidney tubular burden

Western Medicine

Cadmium accumulates primarily in the kidneys and liver, with a biological half-life measured in decades rather than days. Chronic low-level exposure from cigarette smoke, contaminated food, or industrial environments produces gradual kidney tubular damage and mineral dysregulation — often presenting as fatigue, bone density changes, and urinary abnormalities long before blood levels raise concern.

Chinese Medicine

Represents chronic Damp accumulation with progressive Kidney Qi strain. The slow, accumulating nature of cadmium toxicity mirrors the Chinese Medicine understanding of how chronic Damp burdens the Spleen and gradually depletes the Kidney system — the body carrying more than it can process, over a period too long to attribute to any single exposure event.

六邪气 Liù Xié Qì Expression

- Dampness — chronic heaviness, sluggish metabolism, accumulation
- Cold — reduced warmth, metabolic slowing, long-term patterns of depletion

藏象 Zàng Xiàng Involvement

- Kidney — storage, resilience, and long-term recovery capacity
- Spleen — Damp management and transformation

Common Functional Tendencies

- Chronic fatigue with gradual onset
- Cold sensitivity — difficulty maintaining warmth, particularly in the extremities
- Bone or joint discomfort — aching, reduced
- density, or slow healing
- Urinary changes — frequency, nocturia, or reduced concentration capacity
- Reduced resilience and slower recovery from illness or exertion

VOLATILE ORGANIC COMPOUNDS AND ENVIRONMENTAL CHEMICALS

Beyond heavy metals, a growing range of environmental exposure tests measure volatile organic compounds (VOCs) — chemicals that evaporate easily at room temperature and are commonly encountered in daily life. They include gasoline and fuel vapors, paints and solvents, cleaning products, adhesives, and off-gassing from new furniture, carpeting, and building materials. Occupational exposure adds industrial solvents and chemical processing byproducts to this list.

These substances are inhaled through the Lung and processed primarily by the Liver and nervous system. In Western Medicine, repeated exposure may increase metabolic workload and influence nervous system signaling even when standard laboratory tests remain unremarkable — the functional burden precedes measurable structural change.

In Chinese Medicine, VOC exposure patterns are understood through Qi constraint, internal Heat, and Shen disturbance — particularly when ventilation, transformation, or elimination is burdened. The Lung's role as the body's primary environmental boundary makes it the first system to bear the cost of airborne chemical load. When Lung function is strained, the downstream effects include immune sensitivity, skin reactivity, and emotional boundary disruption alongside the more obvious respiratory symptoms.

Common Functional Tendencies in VOC Exposure

Brain fog — Difficulty concentrating, word retrieval problems, mental fatigue disproportionate to activity level

Irritability — Emotional reactivity without clear psychological trigger, particularly after exposure events

Sleep disturbance — Difficulty initiating or maintaining sleep, or unrefreshing sleep

Chemical sensitivity — Heightened reactivity to smells, cleaning products, perfumes, or exhaust

Fatigue after exposure — Energy decline following time in chemically burdened environments — new buildings, recently painted spaces, or high-traffic areas

FUNCTIONAL DISRUPTION APPEARS BEFORE STRUCTURAL CHANGE

The most important clinical principle in this chapter is also the simplest: functional disruption appears before structural change. A patient whose toxicology values are below alert thresholds but whose symptom pattern corresponds precisely to the functional tendencies described above is not imagining their experience. They are in the early stages of a process that laboratory values have not yet fully expressed.

Western toxicology describes what is present. Liù Xiè Qī describes how that presence is expressing as disruption. Zàng Xiàng describes which organ systems are bearing the cost. Together, these frameworks allow a toxicology result to be read as part of a functional picture rather than as an isolated chemical finding.

Exposure Terms — What They Mean Clinically

Detectable — Present at measurable concentrations. Does not indicate injury or disease on its own.

Elevated — Above the population average. Warrants clinical attention and further evaluation of functional impact.

High — Increased burden on the body's clearance and regulatory systems.

Toxic — Functional disruption is present or imminent. The clinical significance is not implied by the number alone — it depends on the pattern of symptoms and system involvement.

Practice makes one thing consistently clear about environmental exposure: the patients most burdened by it are rarely the ones with the highest numbers. They are the ones whose bodies have been compensating quietly for a long time, whose organ systems are bearing a load that the reference range was not designed to detect, and whose symptom patterns tell a story the toxicology report alone cannot fully narrate.

That story is worth telling. This chapter is the framework for reading it.

附章

最佳采血时机

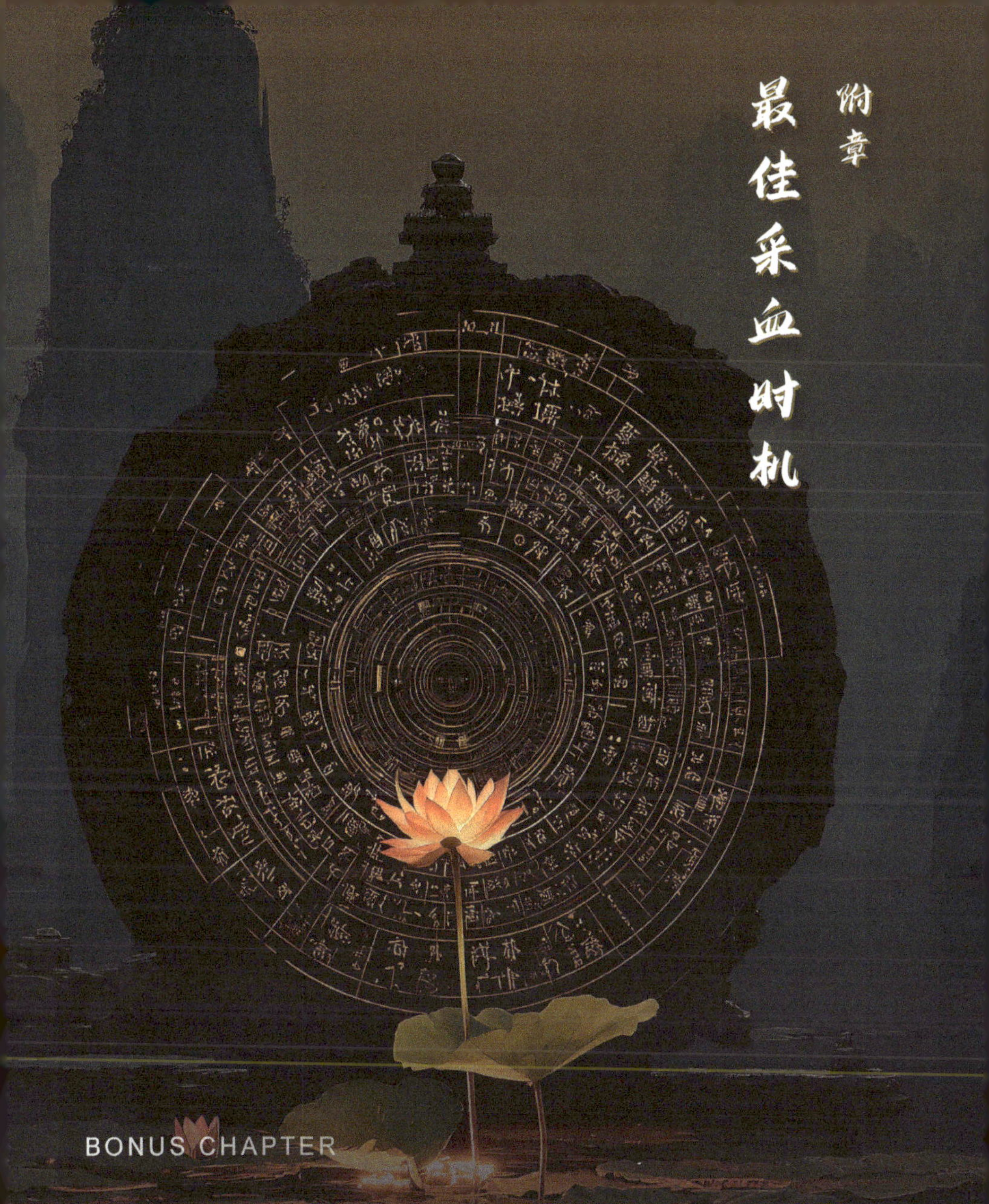

BONUS CHAPTER

When to Draw Blood

HOW TIMING CHANGES EVERYTHING YOUR LAB REPORT SHOWS

When to Draw Blood

HOW TIMING CHANGES EVERYTHING YOUR LAB REPORT SHOWS

There is a question that almost nobody asks — not the physician ordering the test, not the technician drawing the blood, and almost never the patient holding the report. The question is simply this:

> *When was this blood drawn — and what was the body doing at that moment?*

It seems like a small question. It is not. The moment of collection is one of the most consequential variables in laboratory medicine, and it is almost never recorded in a way that informs interpretation. Your report will list your hemoglobin, your cortisol, your glucose, your CRP. It will show you reference ranges. It will flag values that fall outside them. What it will not tell you is whether the timing of the draw captured your body at its peak, its trough, or somewhere in between — and how much that timing shifted the number you are now being asked to interpret.

This chapter exists to close that gap.

The preceding chapters have introduced the idea that blood tests describe a moment rather than a pattern. This chapter takes that idea seriously in a practical direction. It explains what we know — from both Western physiology and classical Chinese Medicine — about how the body's internal clock shapes laboratory values. And it offers something the rest of the book has pointed toward without fully delivering: a working guide to timing-conscious interpretation.

This is not about doubting your laboratory results. It is about reading them with the precision they deserve.

THE BODY IS NOT THE SAME AT EVERY HOUR

Modern physiology has known for decades that the body operates on a 24-hour internal clock — the circadian rhythm. This clock governs almost every measurable biological variable: hormone release, immune activity, body temperature, blood pressure, kidney filtration rate, liver enzyme production, inflammatory signaling, and the concentration of nutrients and metabolites in the blood.

These are not minor fluctuations. Cortisol can vary by a factor of five or six across the day, peaking sharply in the early morning and falling to its lowest point around midnight. Growth hormone, which governs tissue repair and recovery, is released almost entirely during deep sleep, making a morning blood draw nearly useless for assessing it. Melatonin — not just a sleep aid but a potent anti-inflammatory and immune regulator — appears in the blood only after dark and vanishes by dawn. Even iron levels follow a diurnal pattern, typically higher in the morning and lower in the evening, a variation substantial enough to shift interpretation in borderline cases.

The point is not that laboratory tests are unreliable. The point is that they are time-stamped documents from a body in motion. Every value you see on your report was captured at a specific hour, in a specific physiological state, during a specific phase of a cycle that repeats every day. When that context is ignored, the number floats free of meaning. When it is considered, it becomes part of a coherent story.

A Note on Reference Ranges and Timing

Standard reference ranges are derived from population studies in which samples are typically collected in the morning, fasting, under controlled conditions. This means the range printed on your report reflects a morning, fasting body — not your body at 2 PM after a stressful meeting, or at 8 PM when your inflammation may be peaking. A value that appears within range at 8 AM may be meaningfully different at 4 PM, and vice versa. This is not a flaw in laboratory science. It is a context that most lab reports do not explain.

WHAT CHINESE MEDICINE OBSERVED BEFORE THE CLOCK WAS INVENTED

By now the framework introduced at the beginning of this

book — 子午流注 (Zǐ Wǔ Liú Zhù), Midnight-Noon Ebb-Flow — should feel familiar. It has been the lens for every chapter that came before. What the Bonus Chapter offers is a closer look at the structural logic underneath it: why Chinese Medicine recognized the body as a time-ordered system more than two thousand years before modern chronobiology confirmed it, and how that recognition translates into when blood is best drawn.

Zǐ Wǔ Liú Zhù describes the movement of Qì (气) and Xuè (血) through the twelve organ systems in a predictable, time-ordered sequence over the course of a full day and night. Each organ is associated with a two-hour interval — a double-hour (时辰, shí chen) — during which its physiological expression is most pronounced. The body is not running a single rhythm. It is running twelve rhythms in coordinated sequence, and the rhythm of any one organ is most clearly readable inside its own window.

This was not an abstract philosophy. It was a clinical tool. Physicians trained in this system learned to observe not only what a patient presented, but when. A headache that appeared reliably between 11 PM and 1 AM pointed toward a different system than one that arrived each afternoon between 3 and 5 PM. Fatigue that worsened after eating implicated different functional relationships than fatigue that descended at dusk. Timing was diagnostic information — as specific and as actionable as a pulse quality or a tongue presentation.

The body was never understood as a static object to be measured. It was understood as a rhythmic process to be observed over time.

What Zi Wu Liu Zhu teaches — and what modern chronobiology now confirms — is that physiology is not a fixed state. It is a sequence. The body's systems take turns being primary. Organs peak and recede. Inflammatory activity rises and falls. The same molecule measured at different hours carries different clinical meaning. A glucose value in the afternoon is not the same physiological statement as a glucose value at dawn. A cortisol level drawn at noon is not the same signal as one drawn at 8 AM, even if the numbers appear identical.

This matters for how we read blood tests. If every test is drawn at roughly the same hour — as they typically are, in the early morning — we are looking at a single frame from a continuous film. We may be capturing the body's best performance of the day, or its worst, without knowing which.

THE TWELVE-HOUR CYCLE: A REFERENCE GUIDE

The framework introduced at the beginning of this book is the same framework this reference guide rests on. The distinction at its center is worth holding clearly before reading the table.

Meridian Time, the outer ring of the cycle, describes the peak flow of Qi through the surface channel pathways. It is what most online "Chinese Medicine organ clock" charts and popular books display: Gallbladder from 11 PM to 1 AM, Liver from 1 to 3 AM, Lung from 3 to 5 AM. Organ Time, the inner ring, describes when the physical organs themselves are most physiologically active. The two sequences are offset from each other by approximately two hours, and the clinical implications of that offset are significant.

This book uses Organ Time throughout. So does hospital-based Chinese Medicine practice, and so does Western physiology when it tracks circadian rhythms in actual organ function.

The single most instructive example: meridian-based charts assign 11 PM to 1 AM to the Gallbladder. Organ Time assigns that same window to the Kidneys. A patient who wakes consistently between 11 PM and 1 AM with an urge to urinate, a racing heart, or night sweats is not experiencing a gallbladder issue. They are experiencing the Kidneys at peak activity — which Western physiology confirms is exactly when renal filtration, ADH signaling, and adrenal-renal coordination reach their daily expression. Urinalysis and creatinine values drawn in this window reflect actual kidney activity. The pattern is not coincidental. It is anatomical.

The table below uses Organ Time throughout. The biomedical correlations are drawn from the actual organ active in each window — not from the surface meridian passing through it.

THE TWELVE-HOUR ORGAN TIME CYCLE

Organ Time — Biomedical Activity & Laboratory Relevance

Organ Time vs. Meridian Time — Why It Matters

Meridian Time (outer ring) describes the peak flow of Qi through the surface channel pathways — historically used for acupuncture point selection and needle timing. Organ Time (inner ring) describes when the physical organs are most metabolically active — clinically relevant for laboratory interpretation, symptom timing, and biomedical correlation. These two sequences are offset by approximately two hours. When you see an organ clock online, it is almost always the Meridian Time sequence. The Organ Time sequence used in hospital-based clinical practice — and throughout this book — is different, and it is the one that aligns with what blood tests actually measure.

Time | Active Organ (Organ Time)	Biomedical Activity & Laboratory Relevance
11 PM – 1 AM **Kidneys (肾, Shèn)**	The kidneys are at peak filtration and hormonal activity in this window. Renin-angiotensin-aldosterone signaling is active; ADH (antidiuretic hormone) governs water reabsorption. Waking in this window with nocturia, the urge to urinate, is not incidental. It reflects actual renal activity at its peak. Creatinine, BUN, and urinalysis results drawn in this window capture the kidney system at maximum expression. Night sweats, lower back aching, and ankle swelling that occur here are renal-system signals. This is not a Gallbladder hour, despite what most online organ clocks show.

Time | Active Organ (Organ Time)	Biomedical Activity & Laboratory Relevance
1 AM – 3 AM **San Jiao / Triple Burner (三焦, Sān Jiāo)**	The San Jiao governs the coordination of warmth, fluids, and metabolic signaling across the body's three cavities. In Western terms, this maps to the autonomic nervous system's overnight regulatory activity, thermoregulation, fluid redistribution, and the maintenance of homeostasis during deep sleep. Waking in this window with temperature dysregulation, unusual thirst, or a sense of internal restlessness often reflects disruption at this coordinative level rather than any single organ failure. TSH begins its overnight peak in this window.
3 AM – 5 AM **Liver (肝, Gān)**	The liver is actively engaged in detoxification, hormonal clearance, and glycogen regulation between 3 and 5 AM. Cytochrome P450 enzyme activity peaks here; the liver processes the day's metabolic byproducts, clears spent hormones, and releases stored glucose to support the pre-dawn cortisol rise. ALT and AST values, while typically drawn in the morning, reflect the liver's overnight workload. Waking in this window with restlessness, vivid dreams, hot flashes, or hypoglycemic symptoms often indicates the liver is overburdened, by medications, alcohol, hormonal load, or sustained emotional strain.
5 AM – 7 AM **Gallbladder (胆, Dǎn)**	Bile production and release ramp up in preparation for the day's first meal. Fat digestion and cholesterol metabolism become active. This is also when cortisol continues its sharp rise toward its morning peak. Standard blood draws occur in this window or immediately after it, which means most fasting labs are capturing the body as it exits the liver's overnight detoxification phase and enters the gallbladder's digestive preparation phase. Lipid values drawn here reflect this transitional state: storage is shifting toward availability.

Time | Active Organ (Organ Time)	Biomedical Activity & Laboratory Relevance
7 AM – 9 AM **Pericardium (心包, Xīn Bāo)**	The Pericardium governs cardiovascular protection and the interface between the Heart and emotional demand. In Western physiology, this window sees peak cortisol, rising blood pressure and heart rate, and the highest daily incidence of cardiovascular events, myocardial infarction and stroke occur most frequently in the early morning hours. This is not a Stomach hour despite what meridian charts suggest. The cardiovascular system is under its greatest daily strain here. Patients with anxiety, palpitations, or blood pressure instability who report symptoms specifically in the early morning are describing Pericardium-window vulnerability.
9 AM – 11 AM **Small Intestine (小腸, Xiǎo Cháng)**	The small intestine is at peak absorptive and sorting activity. Nutrient assimilation, vitamins, minerals, amino acids, is most efficient in this window. Iron absorption, folate uptake, and fat-soluble vitamin processing are active. From a laboratory perspective, micronutrient values drawn in the late morning may reflect the post-absorptive phase of this window. Persistent cognitive fog, difficulty concentrating, or sensory sensitivity in the mid-morning often reflect Small Intestine sorting dysfunction, the body's inability to efficiently separate what is useful from what should be discarded, both nutritionally and informationally.

Time | Active Organ (Organ Time)	Biomedical Activity & Laboratory Relevance
11 AM – 1 PM **Heart (心, Xīn)**	This is the one window where Organ Time and Meridian Time align. The Heart governs both circulation and mental coherence (Shen, 神). Cardiovascular output is near its daily peak. Blood pressure and heart rate are elevated. Cognitively, this is often the most focused and expressive window of the day. Cardiovascular markers, including troponin in acute settings, are most meaningfully interpreted in the context of this peak demand period. Midday symptoms of palpitations, chest pressure, or cognitive overwhelm are Heart-window presentations.
1 PM – 3 PM **Spleen (脾, Pí)**	The Spleen governs transformation and transportation, the conversion of nutrients into usable Qi and Blood, and their distribution to tissues. In Western physiology, insulin sensitivity begins to decline from its morning peak in this window, and the parasympathetic shift following midday digestion creates the familiar "afternoon slump." Blood sugar regulation is most challenged here. Patients who crash consistently at 1–3 PM, experience post-lunch fatigue, or notice foggy thinking after eating are describing Spleen Qi strain. Fasting glucose and HbA1c do not capture this window; the body's afternoon glucose management is functionally invisible to a morning blood draw.
3 PM – 5 PM **Stomach (胃, Wèi)**	Gastric acid secretion sees a secondary peak in the mid-afternoon. Digestive enzyme activity is elevated. In Western physiology, inflammatory markers, including CRP and histamine, often reach their daily high in this window, and allergic reactivity peaks in the late afternoon for many individuals. This is not a Bladder hour. Patients who experience afternoon acid reflux, food sensitivities, bloating, or inflammatory flares between 3 and 5 PM are experiencing Stomach-window activity. CRP drawn at 8 AM will often appear reassuring for patients whose inflammatory activity peaks in this window, a direct clinical consequence of drawing at the wrong time.

Time | Active Organ (Organ Time)	Biomedical Activity & Laboratory Relevance
5 PM – 7 PM **Lung (肺, Fèi)**	The Lung governs exchange, boundary, and the distribution of Wei Qi (defensive energy) to the body's surface. In Western physiology, respiratory function is near its daily peak in the late afternoon, lung capacity, bronchodilation, and oxygen exchange efficiency are all highest between 4 and 6 PM. This is not a Kidney hour. Patients with asthma or respiratory sensitivity who notice symptoms in this window are expressing Lung-time vulnerability, not renal strain. Pulmonary function tests and peak flow measurements drawn in this window will show different values than those drawn in the early morning, a clinically significant variation for respiratory disease management.
7 PM – 9 PM **Large Intestine (大腸, Dà Cháng)**	The large intestine governs final processing and release. Peristaltic activity continues in the evening, preparing for elimination. In Chinese Medicine, the Large Intestine also governs the release of what no longer serves, physically and emotionally. Constipation, bloating, or difficulty letting go of ruminating thoughts that consistently arise in this window often reflect Large Intestine-time dysregulation. This is not a Pericardium hour.
9 PM – 11 PM **Bladder (膀胸, Páng Guāng)**	The Bladder governs fluid passage and works in functional partnership with the Kidneys. As the body prepares for sleep, the Bladder stores and manages fluid that the kidneys have been processing through the day. Cortisol has reached its daily nadir. Melatonin is rising. In this window, the body should be completing its transition from sympathetic to parasympathetic dominance. Patients who are still alert, anxious, or unable to begin sleep in the 9–11 PM window are resisting the Bladder-time transition, the natural preparation for the Kidney activity that follows at 11 PM. Difficulty with this transition often predicts the nocturia or night waking that follows in the Kidney window.

The table above uses Organ Time throughout. The biomedical correlations are drawn from the actual organ active in each window, not the surface meridian passing through it.

WHAT THIS MEANS FOR YOUR BLOOD TESTS — SPECIFICALLY

Theory becomes useful only when it changes what you do. The following is a practical account of how timing affects the most commonly ordered tests and what it means for interpretation.

Cortisol

Cortisol is the body's primary timing hormone. It should be highest in the first hour after waking — typically 15 to 25 µg/dL — and lowest around midnight, where it may fall below 5 µg/dL. A single cortisol value, drawn at 8 AM without knowledge of when the patient woke, whether they slept well, or how much stress preceded the draw, is of limited interpretive value.

What matters clinically is the curve. A patient with a blunted morning cortisol and elevated evening cortisol will experience fatigue upon waking and wired alertness at night — a pattern that a single morning draw may miss entirely if the morning value happens to appear within range. In Chinese Medicine, this pattern often reflects Kidney Yang depletion with rising Liver Yang — the body's reserves insufficient to power the morning transition, with compensatory agitation emerging in the evening.

Using Organ Time: the pattern of waking exhausted, fighting to rouse until mid-morning, yet feeling alert after 10 PM maps cleanly onto the Kidney-to-San Jiao-to-Liver overnight sequence. The Kidney governs reserve (11 PM–1 AM); the San Jiao governs overnight coordination and thermoregulation (1–3 AM); the Liver governs pre-dawn hormonal clearance and blood sugar release (3–5 AM). A body struggling through these three consecutive windows will experience exactly the morning cortisol pattern described above — because the organs that prepare the body for the cortisol rise are themselves under strain before the morning draw occurs.

Inflammatory Markers (CRP, ESR, Ferritin)

Inflammatory activity is not constant. It follows a diurnal pattern that, in many people, peaks in the late afternoon and evening as the body shifts from output to repair. CRP can vary meaningfully across the day, and ESR — which reflects longer-standing inflammatory viscosity — is influenced by cumulative activity rather than any single moment.

The clinical consequence is this: a CRP drawn at 8 AM in a fasting, resting patient may appear reassuring while the same patient experiences joint stiffness, fatigue, and diffuse aching that intensifies every afternoon. The inflammatory process is real. The blood draw simply did not happen during its most expressive window. This is one of the most common sources of the interpretive gap described in this book.

Using Organ Time correctly: inflammatory symptoms that peak in the 3–5 PM window fall within Stomach time — not Bladder time, as meridian-based charts suggest. This matters because the clinical picture of afternoon inflammation is better understood through gastric and digestive physiology: acid secretion, histamine activity, and food-triggered inflammatory responses are all Stomach-system functions that peak in this window. Evening inflammation and respiratory sensitivity between 5 and 7 PM falls within Lung time — the Lung governs the body's surface boundary and its first-line immune response. When your CRP is drawn at 8 AM and appears normal, but you have daily inflammatory flares at 4 PM, the body is telling you something the morning draw cannot hear.

Thyroid (TSH, Free T4, Free T3)

TSH — the signal the pituitary sends to stimulate thyroid hormone production — follows a clear daily rhythm. It rises in the late evening and early morning hours, peaks around midnight to 2 AM, and reaches its lowest point in the mid-afternoon, typically between 2 and 4 PM. This means that a TSH drawn in the early morning will be higher than one drawn in the afternoon — a difference that can matter when values are borderline.

A patient whose TSH is 3.8 mIU/L at 8 AM might show a TSH of 2.1 mIU/L at 3 PM. Neither value is outside the conventional reference range, but the morning value might prompt a conversation about thyroid support while the afternoon value generates no concern. Same thyroid. Different hour. Different number. Different response.

Free T3 — the active form of thyroid hormone that drives metabolism, temperature, and cognitive speed — also varies, with lower values in the early morning before the day's metabolic demands have ramped up. If you consistently feel cold, slow, and cognitively foggy in the morning despite TSH values that your physician considers normal, the timing of your draw is relevant information.

Glucose and Insulin

Fasting glucose, drawn in the early morning, captures overnight regulation. It is a useful baseline. What it does not capture is how the body manages glucose across the rest of the day — after meals, under stress, during the afternoon cortisol trough, or in the evening when insulin sensitivity declines.

Many patients with perfectly normal fasting glucose experience significant afternoon crashes, post-meal fatigue, and evening cravings that reflect impaired glucose regulation outside the fasting window. In Chinese Medicine, these patterns are understood through the Spleen and Liver systems: the Spleen governs transformation of food into usable energy, while the Liver governs the smooth release of stored energy (glycogen) into the blood. When either system is strained, energy becomes erratic even when fasting numbers appear stable.

Using Organ Time: post-meal crashes and afternoon glucose instability fall squarely within Spleen time (1–3 PM). The Spleen governs the transformation and transportation of acquired essence — the conversion of food into Qi and Blood. When Spleen function is strained, this conversion becomes inefficient and effortful, producing exactly the post-meal fatigue, brain fog, and blood sugar volatility that a morning fasting draw will never capture. The afternoon glucose story is a Spleen story. A morning fasting glucose is not.

Hormones (Estrogen, Progesterone, Testosterone, Hormone D3)

Hormone D3 — commonly and incorrectly labeled as Vitamin D3 — is not a vitamin. It is a hormone, synthesized in the skin from UV light exposure as cholecalciferol, converted by the liver into 25-hydroxyvitamin D (the form most labs actually measure and report), and activated by the kidneys into 1,25-dihydroxyvitamin D (calcitriol) — the form that functions through nuclear receptors to regulate gene expression. I refer to it as the biliary bone matrix hormone precisely because its production pathway runs through cholesterol metabolism and the Liver-Gallbladder system, and its downstream effects govern calcium regulation, immune signaling, and bone mineral density through the Kidney's domain of bone and constitutional reserve. A substance manufactured by the body from sunlight, requiring multi-organ conversion before activation, and governing gene expression through receptor-mediated pathways is, by every definition, a hormone. Labeling it a vitamin has caused it to be underordered, underinterpreted, and disconnected from the hormonal and biliary context where it actually belongs.

Using Organ Time: morning testosterone draws occur during the Pericardium window (7–9 AM) — peak cardiovascular demand, when the body is mobilizing resources for the day. The Pericardium governs the Heart's interface with the external world, which includes the mobilization of Yang energy and its protective expression. This is anatomically consistent with testosterone's role in morning alertness, motivation, and vascular tone. The liver's clearance of sex hormones occurs in its own window (3–5 AM), which means that a borderline testosterone value in the morning may reflect either insufficient production or incomplete overnight clearance — and a morning draw alone cannot distinguish between them.

Iron and Ferritin

Serum iron follows one of the most pronounced diurnal rhythms of any commonly tested value. It is typically 30–50% higher in the morning than in the late afternoon or evening. Ferritin, while more stable, is also influenced by time of day and inflammatory state. A patient who draws blood in the afternoon following a stressful, physically demanding day may show iron levels meaningfully lower than their morning baseline — a variation that could appear as a declining trend if the original draw was done in the morning.

For patients managing iron deficiency, this matters practically. Retesting in the afternoon when the original diagnosis was made from a morning draw may produce numbers that look like improvement or decline, when the variable is actually the hour of collection.

A PRACTICAL FRAMEWORK: READING YOUR REPORT WITH TIMING IN MIND

The following is not a protocol. It is an orientation — a set of questions to bring to your laboratory results and to your clinical conversations.

Before You Interpret a Result, Ask:

1. What time was this blood drawn? Was it consistent with previous draws?
2. What was I doing in the hours before the draw? (Fasting, sleeping, exercising, under stress, already anxious about the appointment?)
3. Does the timing of the draw match the physiological window for this marker? (Cortisol at noon, testosterone at 4 PM, and inflammatory markers at 8 AM will all look different than they would at their respective peaks.)
4. When do my symptoms actually occur? Are they in a different window than when the blood was drawn?
5. Is this a single measurement or part of a trend? If single, what phase of what cycle does it represent?

The gap between when symptoms occur and when blood is drawn is one of the most underappreciated sources of diagnostic confusion in modern medicine. A patient who experiences severe fatigue every afternoon, worsening inflammatory pain each evening, or consistent insomnia between 1 and 3 AM is describing a physiological pattern. When their blood is drawn at 8 AM and returns within normal range, that pattern has not been disproved. It has simply not been measured at the moment of its expression.

Normal at 8 AM does not mean normal at 4 PM. The body did not stop moving while the report was being generated.

This is where the Chinese Medicine framework adds clarity rather than complication. Zi Wu Liu Zhu does not ask you to abandon laboratory medicine. It asks you to treat the timing of your blood draw as clinical data — because it is.

If your persistent symptoms cluster in the late afternoon and your blood is always drawn first thing in the morning, the most important conversation with your physician may not be about your numbers. It may be about requesting a second draw at the time of day when you actually feel unwell. This is not an unreasonable request. It is a precise one.

SYMPTOM TIMING AS DIAGNOSTIC INFORMATION

Classical Chinese Medicine physicians recorded not just what a patient experienced, but when. The reliable appearance of symptoms at particular hours was not considered incidental. It was considered an expression of which system was struggling to complete its cycle.

Modern medicine has mostly discarded this practice. Symptom timing is occasionally documented in specialty settings — gastroenterology, cardiology, sleep medicine — but it is rarely integrated into the interpretation of routine laboratory results. The consequence is a loss of information that costs nothing to collect.

The following correspondences are offered not as diagnoses, but as a starting point for self-observation. If you notice a consistent temporal pattern in your symptoms, that pattern is worth documenting and discussing — alongside, not instead of, your laboratory values.

SYMPTOM TIMING AS DIAGNOSTIC INFORMATION

Organ Time, What Consistent Symptoms at Specific Hours May Reflect

Symptom Timing | Active Organ (Organ Time)	What It Reflects, and Which Lab Values to Consider
9 PM – 11 PM **Bladder**	Difficulty initiating sleep; restlessness; inability to downshift despite exhaustion. The Bladder governs the transition from daytime output to nighttime repair. Resistance here often predicts the nocturia or disrupted sleep that follows in the Kidney window. Consider: urinalysis timing, fluid intake patterns, cortisol nadir.
11 PM – 1 AM **Kidneys**	Waking to urinate (nocturia); night sweats; lower back aching; racing heart or anxiety upon waking. This is active kidney time, the most common window for renal symptoms to surface. Creatinine, BUN, cystatin C, and urinalysis drawn in or near this window capture peak kidney activity. If you consistently wake here and your morning creatinine looks normal, consider whether the draw is timed to the organ's actual peak.
1 AM – 3 AM **San Jiao (Triple Burner)**	Temperature dysregulation, waking too hot or too cold; unusual thirst; sense of internal agitation without clear anxiety. The San Jiao coordinates fluid distribution and thermoregulation across all three body cavities. Disruption here often reflects autonomic dysregulation. TSH peaks during this window; thyroid symptoms that surface overnight may reflect this temporal connection.

Symptom Timing | Active Organ (Organ Time)	What It Reflects, and Which Lab Values to Consider
3 AM – 5 AM **Liver**	Waking with racing thoughts, worry, or vivid disturbing dreams; hot flashes; hypoglycemic sensations (shakiness, sweating, hunger). The liver is actively clearing hormones and regulating blood sugar in this window. ALT, AST, and sex hormone binding globulin values reflect the liver's overnight workload. Persistent waking here, even when liver enzymes appear normal in the morning, often indicates the liver is compensating heavily, from medication burden, hormonal load, or unresolved stress.
5 AM – 7 AM **Gallbladder**	Bitter taste upon waking; right-sided shoulder tension; difficulty making decisions or committing to action upon rising. Bile production is ramping up; cholesterol and fat metabolism are activating. Lipid panels drawn in this window capture the gallbladder's transitional activity. Morning nausea or digestive discomfort here is a Gallbladder-time signal, not a general GI complaint.
7 AM – 9 AM **Pericardium**	Heart palpitations, anxiety, or blood pressure elevation in the early morning; a sense of dread or emotional overwhelm upon waking. This is peak cardiovascular demand time. Morning cardiovascular events, heart attacks, strokes, cluster in this window precisely because the Pericardium is under its greatest daily strain. Morning anxiety that feels disproportionate to circumstances often reflects Pericardium-window vulnerability, not psychological instability.

Symptom Timing | Active Organ (Organ Time)	What It Reflects, and Which Lab Values to Consider
9 AM – 11 AM **Small Intestine**	Cognitive fog, difficulty absorbing or retaining information, sensory overload, or food sensitivity symptoms in the mid-morning. The Small Intestine is sorting and absorbing, nutrients, signals, and experience. Micronutrient deficiencies (iron, B12, folate, fat-soluble vitamins) that persist despite supplementation may reflect Small Intestine sorting dysfunction. Lab values for these markers drawn in this window reflect the post-absorptive phase of peak small intestinal activity.
11 AM – 1 PM **Heart**	Palpitations, chest tightness, or cognitive overload at midday; difficulty maintaining emotional equilibrium under pressure. This is the window where Organ Time and Meridian Time converge. The Heart governs both circulation and Shen (神), mental coherence and presence. Cardiovascular markers are most expressive here. Midday emotional dysregulation often reflects Heart Qi strain rather than psychological weakness.
1 PM – 3 PM **Spleen**	Post-lunch energy crash; brain fog after eating; inability to concentrate in the early afternoon; strong craving for sugar or stimulants. The Spleen governs transformation of food into usable energy. Afternoon glucose instability, not captured by morning fasting draws, is a Spleen-time pattern. HbA1c may appear reassuring while the patient's actual afternoon glucose curve tells a different story.

Symptom Timing | Active Organ (Organ Time)	What It Reflects, and Which Lab Values to Consider
3 PM – 5 PM **Stomach**	Acid reflux, bloating, or digestive discomfort in the mid-afternoon; inflammatory flares, joint stiffness, or histamine reactions peaking between 3 and 5 PM. CRP and ESR drawn at 8 AM regularly appear normal for patients whose inflammatory activity peaks in this Stomach window. If symptoms are consistently in this range and morning markers are clear, an afternoon draw of inflammatory markers may reveal what the standard draw misses.
5 PM – 7 PM **Lung**	Shortness of breath, chest tightness, or skin reactivity in the early evening; grief, sadness, or a sense of unexplained loss at dusk. The Lung governs respiratory exchange and boundary, including the skin and immune surface. Pulmonary function tests in this window will show different values than morning tests. Patients who manage asthma or allergies should note whether symptoms peak here, as this is actual Lung time, not the Kidney hour that meridian charts suggest.
7 PM – 9 PM **Large Intestine**	Evening constipation, bloating, or difficulty fully eliminating; ruminating thoughts that are hard to release; a sense of being unable to "let go" of the day. The Large Intestine governs release, physical and emotional. This is not the Pericardium window that meridian charts assign here.

These correspondences are offered as a starting point for self-observation, not as diagnoses. Always bring consistent temporal symptom patterns to a qualified healthcare professional.

These are not prescriptions. They are patterns — recurring correspondences between time and physiology that two medical traditions, developed independently on opposite sides of the world, both identified as clinically meaningful. When your symptom pattern and your laboratory results seem to tell different stories, timing may be the chapter that connects them.

A WORD ON SEASONAL AND CYCLICAL VARIATION

The body's internal clock operates on more than a 24-hour cycle. Physiology is also governed by seasonal rhythms — shifts in light exposure, temperature, and environmental demand that influence hormone production, immune activity, inflammatory thresholds, and metabolic rate in measurable ways.

Hormone D3, whose role extends well beyond bone health into immune regulation and inflammatory modulation, declines significantly through winter in northern latitudes. Thyroid activity tends to be more robust in cooler months and more restrained in summer — a seasonal adaptation that may explain why some patients feel their symptoms worsen in spring and summer despite identical laboratory values. Inflammatory conditions often flare at seasonal transitions, not only because of allergen exposure, but because the body's regulatory systems are recalibrating their baseline.

The menstrual cycle is another form of temporal variation

with direct laboratory implications. As noted above, hormone values must be interpreted in the context of cycle day. But the menstrual cycle also influences inflammatory markers, thyroid sensitivity, iron levels, and immune activity in ways that a single draw cannot capture. Women who notice predictable symptom patterns at particular cycle phases — premenstrual inflammatory flares, mid-cycle fatigue, post-ovulatory mood changes — are observing real physiology. That observation is laboratory-relevant, even when the standard draw does not coincide with the symptomatic phase.

In Chinese Medicine, this is understood through the rhythm of Yin and Yang across the lunar and seasonal cycles. Yin peaks in winter and at mid-cycle; Yang peaks in summer and at ovulation. When these cycles are dysregulated — by chronic stress, insufficient sleep, irregular schedules, or sustained physiological demand — the body's ability to make each transition gracefully is compromised. Laboratory values may appear stable while the patient experiences increasingly erratic symptoms between draws.

WHAT TIMING-CONSCIOUS INTERPRETATION ACTUALLY LOOKS LIKE

It does not require a different laboratory. It does not require a dozen draws at different hours of the day, though that level of investigation is sometimes warranted. It requires, first and most practically, treating the time of draw as a documented variable rather than an afterthought.

When you receive a laboratory report, note the collection time. Consider whether it aligns with your symptom pattern. If your most significant symptoms occur in a window that your standard morning draw does not capture, say so. Ask whether an additional draw at a different hour might be informative. Bring your symptom timing pattern — not just the symptoms themselves, but when they reliably appear — to your clinical conversations.

This is not alternative medicine. It is precision medicine, applied to a variable that standard laboratory practice has historically undervalued in the West — despite centuries of clinical application in the East.

A Practical Note for Clinical Conversations

When discussing your laboratory results with a physician, consider saying: "I notice my symptoms are consistently worse in the [afternoon/ evening / early morning]. My blood is usually drawn first thing in the morning. Is there value in repeating specific markers at the time when my symptoms are most active?" This is a reasonable, specific, and clinically grounded question. Most physicians will engage with it. Those trained in integrative or functional medicine will recognize it immediately. Even those who are not may find it opens a more useful conversation than simply asking why the numbers look normal when you feel unwell.

The title of this book is The Missing Half of Your Blood Test. Timing is not the only missing half — context, pattern, and functional interpretation all contribute. But timing may be the most practically recoverable piece of missing information. It is, quite literally, something that could be noted on every laboratory requisition at no additional cost, requiring only the awareness that the moment of measurement is part of the measurement.

> *Your blood was drawn at a specific hour. Your body was doing something specific at that hour. Both of those facts belong in the interpretation.*

Zi Wu Liu Zhu — the classical framework that opened this book — is not a clock you follow with mechanical precision. It is a way of understanding that the body has its own sequence, its own rhythm, its own logic of when things happen and why. That understanding does not belong to Chinese Medicine alone. It belongs to anyone who has ever noticed that they feel worse at a particular time of day, and wondered whether the blood test taken at a different hour was telling the whole story.

It was not. This chapter was the rest of it.

后记
词汇表
参考指南

BACK MATTER

Glossary & Reference Guide

A PLAIN-LANGUAGE COMPANION TO READING BLOOD TESTS, BODY PATTERNS, AND CLINICAL LANGUAGE

Glossary & Reference Guide

A PLAIN-LANGUAGE COMPANION TO READING BLOOD TESTS, BODY PATTERNS, AND CLINICAL LANGUAGE

This glossary exists because most people are asked to interpret medical language without being taught the language first. Laboratory tests, toxicology reports, and clinical explanations use words that sound precise but are rarely defined in a way that helps patients understand what is actually being described.

This is not a diagnostic tool. It does not replace clinical care. Its purpose is orientation — understanding what is being measured, what is not being measured, and how Western Medicine and Chinese Medicine describe the same body in different but complementary terms.

You are not meant to read this from beginning to end. Return to it when something feels unfamiliar, when a word on a report raises a question, or when a clinical term needs a plain-language translation.

SECTION A – WESTERN MEDICAL, LAB & TOXICOLOGY TERMS

What blood tests and reports are actually describing.

Core Lab Concepts

Blood Test / Lab Test

A measurement taken from your blood at one specific moment. It shows what was present in your bloodstream at that time – not how your body functions day to day, not how hard it is working to maintain those values, and not what the values look like at a different hour.

Reference Range

The printed interval labeled "normal" on your report. It is based on population averages, not personal health or optimal function. Being within range means your value falls where most people's values fall – not that your body is maintaining that value with ease.

Normal

A value inside the reference range. Normal means common, not necessarily healthy or effortless. A normal value can still reflect significant compensatory effort.

Abnormal / Flagged

A value outside the reference range. It signals statistical difference from the population average, not automatic disease or emergency. A flag calls for closer attention and correlation — not panic.

Biomarker

Any measurable substance or indicator in the body that provides information about biological activity — hormones, enzymes, minerals, inflammatory proteins, or metabolic byproducts.

Baseline

Your usual value when things are stable. Changes from your personal baseline can carry clinical meaning even when values remain within the population reference range.

Variability

Natural fluctuation in values caused by stress, sleep quality, food intake, illness, exercise, hydration, time of day, or menstrual cycle timing. Variability is why a single draw is often insufficient for a complete clinical picture.

Snapshot

A single measurement taken at one moment. Most laboratory tests are snapshots, not continuous monitoring. They describe what was present when the needle went in, not what was present an hour earlier or later.

Trend

A pattern observed when the same test is repeated over time. Trends often carry more clinical meaning than single results — particularly when values move consistently in one direction while remaining within reference range.

False Negative

A test result that appears normal even though strain, dysfunction, or pathology is present. This can occur when blood is drawn outside the window in which a problem is most expressive, or when the marker being measured does not reflect the layer where the problem is occurring.

False Positive

A test result that appears abnormal even though no meaningful problem exists. Can result from testing conditions, timing, laboratory variation, or transient physiological states.

Sensitivity

How well a test detects change when change is genuinely present. A highly sensitive test produces few false negatives.

Specificity

How well a test avoids false alarms. A highly specific test produces few false positives.

Clinical Significance

Whether a result meaningfully affects function or health — not just whether it is statistically different from the population average. A value can be statistically abnormal without being clinically significant, and clinically significant without being statistically flagged.

Statistical Significance

A mathematical difference that exceeds a predefined threshold. Statistical significance does not automatically equal clinical significance.

Blood, Oxygen & Cell Markers

Hemoglobin

A protein in red blood cells that carries oxygen to tissues. The primary marker for anemia assessment.

Hematocrit

The percentage of blood volume made up of red blood cells. Rises and falls in proportion to hemoglobin.

Red Blood Cell Count (RBC)

The number of oxygen-carrying cells per unit of blood. Used alongside hemoglobin and hematocrit to assess oxygen delivery capacity.

White Blood Cell Count (WBC)

The number of immune cells in the blood. Elevated counts suggest active immune response or inflammation; suppressed counts may indicate bone marrow strain or immune compromise.

Platelets

Cell fragments involved in clotting and tissue repair. Low counts suggest bleeding risk; elevated counts may reflect inflammatory activity.

Mean Corpuscular Volume (MCV)

The average size of red blood cells. Smaller than normal suggests iron deficiency or thalassemia; larger than normal suggests B12 or folate deficiency.

Red Cell Distribution Width (RDW)

How much red blood cell size varies within a sample. Greater variation can reflect nutritional deficiency, inflammatory strain, or adaptation.

Metabolism & Energy

Glucose (Fasting)

Blood sugar measured after not eating, used to assess baseline energy regulation. Reflects overnight hepatic regulation

— not how glucose is managed after meals or under stress.

Hemoglobin A1c (HbA1c)

An estimate of average blood sugar over approximately three months. Provides longer-term context that a single fasting glucose cannot.

Insulin

A hormone that moves glucose into cells for energy use. Insulin levels reflect how hard the body is working to manage blood sugar.

Insulin Resistance

A state where cells respond less efficiently to insulin, requiring increased output to maintain normal blood sugar. Often present for years before glucose values become abnormal.

Metabolic Function

How efficiently the body produces, distributes, and uses energy across its various systems.

Metabolic Flexibility

The body's ability to shift between energy sources — glucose and fat — depending on demand and availability.

Lipids & Cardiovascular Markers

Cholesterol

A building material used by the body to produce hormones, maintain cell membranes, insulate nerves, and repair tissue. Not inherently harmful — essential to normal physiology.

LDL (Low-Density Lipoprotein)

A transport particle that carries cholesterol from the liver to tissues requiring it. Elevated LDL may reflect increased repair demand, inflammatory burden, or impaired clearance — not excess alone.

HDL (High-Density Lipoprotein)

A transport particle that returns cholesterol from peripheral tissues to the liver for reuse or elimination. Higher levels generally reflect efficient metabolic recycling.

Triglycerides

A form of stored energy circulating in the blood. Elevated levels are commonly associated with insulin resistance, disrupted sleep, and metabolic overload.

Lipoprotein Particle

The carrier vehicle that moves lipid material through the bloodstream. Particle size and number provide more clinical information than cholesterol content alone.

Cardiovascular Risk Marker

A value used to estimate strain on the heart and blood vessels based on population-level correlations. Reflects probability, not certainty.

Liver, Kidney & Metabolic Markers

ALT (Alanine Aminotransferase)

An enzyme primarily associated with liver cell activity. Elevations reflect liver workload or cellular stress. Persistent high-normal values may indicate constrained Liver function even without a diagnostic flag.

AST (Aspartate Aminotransferase)

An enzyme found in the liver, heart, and skeletal muscle. Elevated alongside ALT suggests liver involvement; elevated without ALT elevation may suggest muscle or cardiac source.

Alkaline Phosphatase (ALP)

An enzyme involved in bile flow and bone metabolism. Elevated values may reflect biliary obstruction, bone turnover, or liver stress.

Bilirubin

A breakdown product of red blood cells processed by the liver. Elevated values may reflect hemolysis, liver dysfunction, or biliary impairment.

Albumin

A protein produced by the liver that maintains fluid balance and transports substances through the blood. Low albumin indicates reduced liver synthetic capacity.

Creatinine

A waste product produced by muscle metabolism and filtered by the kidneys. Rising creatinine, even within range, may indicate declining kidney reserve.

BUN (Blood Urea Nitrogen)

A marker related to protein metabolism and kidney filtration efficiency. Interpreted alongside creatinine to assess kidney function.

GFR (Glomerular Filtration Rate)

An estimate of how efficiently the kidneys filter blood, calculated from creatinine and other factors. Declining GFR over time is clinically significant even when individual values remain within range.

Electrolytes (Sodium, Potassium, Chloride, Bicarbonate)

Minerals that regulate fluid balance, nerve conduction, muscle contraction, and acid-base balance. Even borderline values may carry functional significance.

Inflammation & Immune Markers

Inflammation

The body's response to stress, injury, infection, or irritation. A necessary biological process with distinct phases — protective, resolving, or lingering. Not a disease in itself.

Chronic Inflammation

Low-grade inflammation that persists beyond the acute phase, often without obvious cause. Associated with fatigue, pain, hormonal disruption, and metabolic strain.

CRP (C-Reactive Protein)

A protein produced by the liver in response to inflammatory signaling. Rises quickly with acute inflammation and falls as it resolves. A useful marker for acute events; less reliable for low-grade or time-of-day-variable inflammation.

High-Sensitivity CRP (hs-CRP)

A more sensitive version of the CRP test, capable of detecting low-grade inflammatory activity that standard CRP may not register.

ESR (Erythrocyte Sedimentation Rate)

A measure of how rapidly red blood cells settle in a test tube. Rises more slowly than CRP and reflects longer-standing inflammatory activity.

Ferritin

A protein that stores iron. Also functions as an acute-phase reactant — elevated ferritin may reflect inflammatory or liver stress even when iron stores are not excessive.

Hormones

Hormone D3

Synthesized in the skin as cholecalciferol, converted by the liver into 25-hydroxyvitamin D (the form measured on most lab reports), and activated by the kidneys into 1,25-dihydroxyvitamin D (calcitriol), its biologically active form. Governs calcium metabolism, immune regulation, inflammatory signaling, and bone mineral density.

TSH (Thyroid-Stimulating Hormone)

A signal produced by the pituitary gland to stimulate thyroid hormone production. Reflects regulatory effort rather than output. Follows a diurnal rhythm — highest around midnight, lowest in the mid-afternoon.

Free T4 (Thyroxine)

The reserve form of thyroid hormone. Must be converted to Free T3 to become metabolically active.

Free T3 (Triiodothyronine)

The active form of thyroid hormone that drives metabolism,

temperature regulation, and cognitive speed. Low-normal Free T3 with adequate TSH and T4 suggests a conversion problem rather than a production problem.

Cortisol

A timing and stress-response hormone that should peak in the morning and decline across the day. Rhythm matters as much as quantity — a within-range morning value does not confirm a healthy daily curve.

Toxicology & Environmental Exposure

Toxicology

The study of how substances affect biological systems — their mechanisms, concentrations, and effects on physiology.

Toxin

Any substance that disrupts normal physiological function at sufficient concentration or duration of exposure.

Environmental Exposure

Contact with chemicals or pollutants from air, food, water, products, or occupational settings.

Heavy Metals

Elements such as lead, mercury, arsenic, and cadmium that interfere with neurological, immune, and metabolic function. Effects are often cumulative and gradual.

Bioaccumulation

The gradual buildup of substances in body tissues over time, particularly when clearance is slower than intake.

Body Burden

The total accumulation of environmental chemicals stored in the body at any given time.

Exposure vs. Toxicity

A detectable level of a substance indicates presence. It does not automatically indicate injury or disease. Toxicity describes functional disruption — which depends on concentration, duration, form, and individual system response.

Clearance

The body's ability to process and eliminate substances over time. Impaired clearance — from liver strain, nutritional depletion, or genetic variation — increases body burden even at moderate exposure levels.

Half-Life

The time required for half of a substance to be eliminated from the body. Half-lives vary widely: hours for some compounds, decades for others (such as cadmium in kidney tissue).

Synergistic Effects

When multiple exposures together produce a stronger effect than any single exposure alone. Combined burdens can exceed what the body's clearance systems can manage efficiently.

SECTION B — CLASSICAL CHINESE MEDICINE TERMS

How Chinese Medicine describes the body, its functions, and its patterns of health and imbalance.

The 黄帝内经 — 素问 (Huángdì Nèijīng — Sù Wèn), the foundational classical text of Chinese Medicine, describes the body as a living system that must move, warm, nourish, rest, and recover in rhythm with life. Health is not defined by isolated numbers. It is defined by whether the body can respond to stress, digest and assimilate nourishment, circulate blood and warmth, rest and recover, and maintain balance over time. Organs are not described as mechanical parts. They are described by their responsibilities.

Fundamental Concepts

Qi — 气 (Qì)

The body's capacity to do work or act. Not a substance — the activity behind every process: moving blood, digesting food, generating warmth, thinking clearly, responding to stress, repairing tissue. When Qi is sufficient and flowing, life feels manageable. When Qi is weak, scattered, or stuck, everything requires more effort.

Blood — 血 (Xué)

What nourishes and anchors life. Beyond carrying oxygen, Blood provides moisture, stability, grounding, and mental calm. When Blood is insufficient or poorly circulated, the body may feel dry, restless, weak, cold, or unsteady — even when laboratory values appear normal. Qi moves Blood; Blood nourishes Qi.

Yin — 阴 (Yīn)

The cooling, nourishing, containing, and restorative aspect of physiology. Substance, moisture, rest, repair, and storage. When Yin is depleted, the body overheats, dries, and cannot sustain the rest and recovery it needs.

Yang — 阳 (Yáng)

The warming, activating, and mobilizing aspect of physiology. Warmth, movement, activity, and output. When Yang is deficient, the body slows, cools, and cannot generate the energy and initiative daily function requires.

Jing — 精 (Jīng)

Deep constitutional reserve stored by the Kidneys. The body's long-term endowment — the capacity for sustained effort, recovery from illness, endurance, and graceful aging.

Depletes slowly over a lifetime; laboratory markers often lag behind its decline.

Shen — 神 (Shén)

Mental coherence, consciousness, and the quality of presence. Governed by the Heart. When Shen is settled, the mind is clear and the person feels integrated. When Shen is disturbed, restlessness, anxiety, sleep disruption, and emotional instability follow.

Organ Systems — Zang (Storage) Organs

The Zang organs store essential substances and preserve physiological function over time. They are described by what they are responsible for, not only what they contain.

Liver — 肝 (Gān)

Governs smooth movement — the free circulation of Qi and Blood, the smooth processing of emotional experience, and the body's adaptation to stress. When Liver function is strained: tension, irritability, pressure sensations, symptoms that come and go unpredictably, and difficulty winding down.

Heart — 心 (Xīn)

Governs circulation and coherence. Blood moves rhythmically, warmth reaches tissues, and the mind feels settled and clear. The Heart is also associated with consciousness and integration (Shen). When Heart function is disturbed: restlessness, palpitations, poor sleep, difficulty settling mentally.

Spleen — 脾 (Pí)

Governs transformation and transportation — converting food and experience into usable Qi and Blood, and distributing nourishment throughout the body. When Spleen function is weak: fatigue, bloating, foggy thinking, a sense of heaviness, and difficulty converting food into sustained energy.

Lung — 肺 (Fèi)

Governs exchange and boundaries — bringing in fresh air, distributing fluids and nourishment, releasing what is no longer needed. Also governs immunity and the skin. When Lung function is strained: respiratory sensitivity, reduced resistance to illness, skin reactivity, or difficulty with emotional boundaries.

Kidney — 肾 (Shèn)

Stores deep reserves (Jing). Governs growth, development, aging, recovery capacity, and endurance. The foundation of long-term vitality. When Kidney reserves are depleted: chronic tiredness, slow recovery, cold sensitivity below the waist, low back soreness, and a sense of premature aging.

Pericardium — 心包 (Xīn Bāo)

The Heart's protector. Buffers emotional shock, stress, and overstimulation. When overwhelmed: emotional sensitivity, shutdown, or protective withdrawal — even when the Heart itself is intact.

Organ Systems — Fu (Hollow) Organs

The Fu organs process and move. They do not store — they receive, transform, and pass along.

Stomach — 胃 (Wèi)

Receives food and drink and initiates breakdown. The beginning of the digestive process. When weak: discomfort, inefficient digestion, acid reflux, or nausea — particularly in the Organ Time window of 3–5 PM.

Small Intestine — 小肠 (Xiǎo Cháng)

Sorts and separates the useful from the unusable — nutritionally and, metaphorically, informationally. Governs assimilation of nourishment. When strained: poor nutrient absorption, cognitive difficulty, sensory overload.

Large Intestine — 大肠 (Dà Cháng)

Governs release — the final elimination of waste after nourishment has been extracted. Also associated with the ability to let go emotionally. When strained: constipation, bloating, difficulty with endings or release.

Gallbladder — 胆 (Dǎn)

Supports decision-making, direction, and the capacity to commit to action. Works closely with the Liver in governing movement and bile production. When strained: hesitation, indecision, difficulty initiating.

Urinary Bladder — 膀胱 (Páng Guāng)

Manages fluid passage and elimination in partnership with the Kidneys. The final stage of fluid regulation. Active in the Organ Time window of 9–11 PM — the body's transition into overnight repair.

San Jiao / Triple Burner — 三焦 (Sān Jiāo)

Coordinates the movement of warmth, fluids, and signals across the body's three cavities (upper, middle, and lower). Has no physical organ form — describes communication and distribution between systems. Active in the Organ Time window of 1–3 AM.

Functional Patterns

These describe how imbalance appears in the body — not diagnoses in the Western sense, but clinical patterns that organize symptoms and guide interpretation.

Qi Stagnation — 气滞 (Qì Zhì)

Qi is present but not moving freely. Often felt as tension, pressure, irritability, or symptoms that are better with movement and worse with prolonged stillness.

Blood Stasis — 血瘀 (Xuè Yū)

Blood is present but circulation is impaired. Often felt as fixed pain, dark complexion, slow healing, or clotting tendencies.

Deficiency — 虚 (Xū)

Insufficient capacity to meet physiological demands. Often felt as fatigue, weakness, pallor, or reduced resilience. Deficiency of Qi, Blood, Yin, or Yang each produces a distinct clinical picture.

Excess — 实证 (Shí Zhèng)

Too much accumulation or obstruction. Often felt as fullness, agitation, pain with pressure, or a sense of blockage that does not resolve with rest.

Heat — 热 (Rè)

Processes are too active or too hot. Often felt as inflammation, restlessness, thirst, or heat sensations — particularly in the evening when Yin should be rising to contain Yang.

Cold — 寒 (Hán)

Processes are too slow or too cold. Often felt as coldness, low energy, slow digestion, or reduced motivation.

Dampness — 湿 (Shī)

Fluids are not moving and transforming efficiently. Often felt as heaviness, fogginess, bloating, or a sense of being weighed down.

Constraint — 郁 (Yù)

Normal expression is suppressed or held back — often from prolonged emotional stress, unresolved experience, or sustained demands without sufficient release.

Diagnostic Frameworks

Ba Gang — 八纲 (Bā Gāng): The Eight Principles

The foundational diagnostic framework organizing clinical findings into four pairs: Yin/Yang, Excess/Deficiency, Heat/Cold, Interior/Exterior. These pairs describe the nature and location of imbalance, guiding appropriate clinical response.

Zang Xiang — 藏象 Zàng Xiàng

Means "how the organs show themselves." Rather than asking whether an organ is damaged, this system asks whether its function is expressed clearly and its role fulfilled over time. Organs can be strained long before structural disease appears.

Liu Xie Qi — 六邪气 (Liù Xié Qì): The Six Excesses

Wind, Cold, Heat, Dampness, Dryness, and Summer-Heat. Describes how environmental or internal disruption expresses in the body, regardless of its original cause. Environmental exposure, emotional strain, and physiological depletion can all produce Six Excess patterns.

Si Zhen — 四诊 (Sì Zhěn): The Four Examinations

The four primary clinical assessment methods: looking (望, wàng), listening and smelling (闻, wén), asking (问, wèn), and touching (切, qiē). Laboratory values clarify and confirm what the Four Examinations have already observed. They do not replace clinical observation.

SECTION C — TIME, RHYTHM & CONTEXT

Why when a test is taken changes what it shows — and what timing reveals that numbers alone cannot.

Circadian Rhythm

The body's internal 24-hour clock. Governs hormones, temperature, energy, digestion, immune activity, and virtually every measurable physiological variable. Because of circadian rhythm, the same test taken at different hours can produce meaningfully different values — without any change in the underlying condition.

Zi Wu Liu Zhu — 子午流注 (Zǐ Wǔ Liú Zhù)

Midnight-Noon Ebb-Flow. The classical Chinese Medicine framework describing how physiological activity moves through the body in a predictable, time-ordered sequence across the 24-hour cycle. Each organ system has a period of peak activity. The timing of blood collection, symptoms, and interventions is understood in relation to this cycle.

Organ Time (Inner Ring)

The clinical timing sequence used in hospital-based Chinese Medicine practice and throughout this book. Describes when the physical organs themselves are most metabolically and physiologically active. This sequence is offset from the more commonly circulated Meridian Time sequence by approximately two hours. Organ Time aligns with Western physiological data on organ activity across the day.

Meridian Time (Outer Ring)

The timing sequence describing peak Qi flow through the surface channel (meridian) pathways — historically used for acupuncture point selection and needle timing. The sequence most commonly found in online organ clock resources. Distinct from Organ Time and not used as the basis for laboratory interpretation in this book.

Diurnal Variation

Normal day-night fluctuation in physiological values. Many body markers shift meaningfully across the day because the body is designed to shift. Diurnal variation is why cortisol, testosterone, TSH, iron, and inflammatory markers can look different depending on collection time.

Timing Mismatch

When a test is taken at a time that does not correspond to the body's natural peak or trough for that function. Can cause a result to appear normal when the problem occurs at a different hour, or abnormal when the value was captured at a transient peak.

Testing Conditions

The full circumstances surrounding a blood draw: fasting status, sleep quality, stress level, exercise in the preceding hours, hydration, time of day, menstrual cycle timing, and medications or supplements. Testing conditions influence results significantly and are often not recorded on laboratory reports.

Baseline vs. Peak vs. Recovery

Three distinct physiological states that a single draw may capture without indicating which one. Baseline is the resting state. Peak is the stress or demand state. Recovery is the return toward baseline. A normal result in a recovery state does not mean the peak was also normal.

Seasonal Variation

Physiological shifts that correspond to seasonal changes in light exposure, temperature, and environmental demand. Affects immune function, Hormone D3 levels, thyroid activity, mood, and inflammatory thresholds. A single annual draw does not capture seasonal variation.

Symptom Timing Pattern

A pattern in which symptoms appear consistently at a specific time of day — morning fatigue, afternoon crashes, evening inflammation, early-morning waking. Symptom timing patterns often provide clearer diagnostic information than isolated laboratory values, particularly in the gray zone between normal and abnormal.

SECTION D — INTEGRATIVE & INTERPRETIVE TERMS

The bridge language that connects laboratory numbers to lived experience — without making claims the data cannot support.

Interpretive Gap

The space between what laboratory results show and how the body actually feels. Exists because tests measure certain things well but do not measure everything that generates fatigue, pain, fog, mood changes, or weakness. The interpretive gap is why someone can feel consistently unwell with results that appear normal.

Interpretive Mismatch

When results suggest stability but symptoms suggest strain — or when symptoms improve but laboratory values have not yet shifted. A mismatch does not mean symptoms are imaginary. It means the test may not be measuring the most relevant layer, or that the body's functional recovery is preceding its biochemical recovery.

Pattern

A repeated relationship observed over time — symptom timing, recurring borderline values, consistent crashes after stress, or fluctuating markers. Patterns carry more clinical information than single results because the body is dynamic, not static.

Snapshot Bias

Over-reliance on a single laboratory result. A snapshot can miss problems that fluctuate, depend on timing, or only appear under conditions of stress or demand.

Temporal Context

Understanding a value within its timing — time of day, stage of stress, stage of recovery, and relevant recent history. Temporal context is what turns a number into meaningful clinical information.

Contextual Interpretation

Reading results within real-life conditions: sleep, stress,

diet, activity, hydration, cycle timing, medications, and symptoms. Context does not excuse a result — it explains it.

Compensated Normal

A state in which laboratory values appear normal only because the body is expending significant effort to maintain them. This concept explains the common experience of being told "you're fine" while lived experience consistently suggests otherwise.

Functional Stability

Stability that exists numerically but not experientially. Values are in range; function does not feel stable. Functional stability can mask an approaching threshold where compensatory capacity finally runs out.

Hidden Strain

Physiological load that does not show clearly on standard tests. May appear as reduced resilience, delayed recovery, frequent crashes, poor sleep quality, or growing sensitivity to stressors that were previously tolerable.

Functional Expression

How the body shows its internal state in daily life: energy, mood, digestion, sleep quality, temperature regulation, motivation, recovery time, and mental clarity. Often the most honest available report of what is actually happening.

Regulation

The ability to respond appropriately to demand and return to baseline. Good regulation means stress is tolerated and recovery follows. Poor regulation means small stressors produce disproportionate consequences and recovery is slow.

Regulatory Bandwidth

The range of demand the body can handle before symptoms appear. Wide bandwidth allows tolerance of stress without consequence. Narrowed bandwidth means small disruptions become significant.

Reserve

Stored physiological capacity — what the body draws on when it works late, misses sleep, gets ill, or goes through sustained emotional strain. People can function apparently well for years while spending reserve, until it runs low.

Adaptive Reserve

How much reserve remains available. When adaptive reserve is depleted, symptoms become more frequent, more intense, and recovery takes longer. Restoring capacity is often more clinically important than treating individual symptoms.

Distribution

Whether resources present in the blood are actually reaching the tissues that need them. A value can appear adequate in the blood while delivery to target tissues is impaired.

Distribution Failure

Resources exist but delivery is disrupted — by stress physiology, inflammation, circulation impairment, or timing mismatch. One reason laboratory values can appear normal while functional capacity is not.

Tissue Availability

Whether a substance present in the blood is usable at the tissue level. Blood values do not automatically equal tissue function.

Demand vs. Supply

A simple model: the body has needs (demand) and resources (supply). Problems emerge when demand rises too high, supply drops too low, or delivery between the two breaks down.

Transformation

The conversion of inputs into usable function — food into energy, thyroid hormone into active form, rest into recovery. Transformation can fail even when the inputs are adequate.

Transformation Failure

Inputs are present but conversion is impaired. A patient may eat sufficiently and still feel depleted if the Spleen's transforming function is weak, or have adequate T4 and still feel hypothyroid if T4-to-T3 conversion is inefficient.

Signal vs. Output

A signal is a message (hormone, nerve cue, enzyme activation). Output is what happens in the target tissue in response. A signal can appear normal while output is impaired — or a signal may be elevated because the body is compensating for insufficient output.

Root vs. Branch

Root is the underlying condition generating the problem. Branch is the symptom or abnormal marker that the root produces. Treating the branch may relieve symptoms temporarily; addressing the root improves long-term stability.

Surface vs. Depth

Surface is what is visible now — a symptom, a flagged value. Depth refers to underlying reserve, regulation, and capacity. Depth explains why surface problems recur.

Storage vs. Circulation

Having resources and moving them are two different functions. Adequate storage with impaired circulation still produces functional deficiency at the tissue level.

Nourishment

Long-term tissue support — what actually reaches tissues and restores them. Not only food, but sleep, digestion, blood flow, hydration, minerals, and recovery. Nourishment is the cumulative result of all of these functioning well together.

Warming Function

The body's ability to generate energy and warmth — physically (temperature regulation) and functionally (motivation, digestion, circulation). Associated with Yang in Chinese Medicine.

Cooling Function

The body's ability to calm excess activity, reduce inflammation, quiet agitation, and prevent overactivation. Associated with Yin in Chinese Medicine.

Manifestation

How internal states show up outwardly — through symptoms, laboratory values, sleep patterns, mood, or timing patterns. The visible report of deeper processes.

Framework

A structured way of understanding what is being observed. A framework helps ask better questions rather than chasing individual explanations. Both Western laboratory medicine and Chinese Medicine are frameworks — each with its own design, its own strengths, and its own blind spots.

Model Limitation

Every interpretive model has blind spots. Laboratory models, pattern models, and clinical frameworks alike. Knowing the limitations of a model prevents overconfidence and supports more accurate interpretation.

Observation vs. Explanation

Observation is what can be seen or measured — a number, a symptom, a pattern. Explanation is why it is occurring. Keeping these distinct is how interpretation stays honest.

Orientation

Knowing what kind of information you are looking at, what it can tell you, and what it cannot. Orientation reduces alarm and confusion. It is the goal of this entire book.

Over-interpretation

Assigning more meaning to a result than the evidence supports. Over-interpretation increases fear and leads to pursuing noise rather than signal.

Clarity

Understanding without oversimplification. Feeling more oriented rather than more alarmed. The condition this book aims to produce in every reader who reaches this page.

In the 黄帝内经 Huángdì Nèijīng, health is not perfection. It is responsiveness.

This language exists to describe how life flows — or fails to flow — through the body over time, often long before laboratory values change. The terms in this glossary are not a vocabulary to be memorized. They are tools for asking better questions, having clearer conversations, and understanding your own physiology with the steadiness that comes from orientation rather than alarm.

关于作者

ABOUT THE AUTHOR

Dr. Kamal Polite

DCEM, DOM, AP, CHE

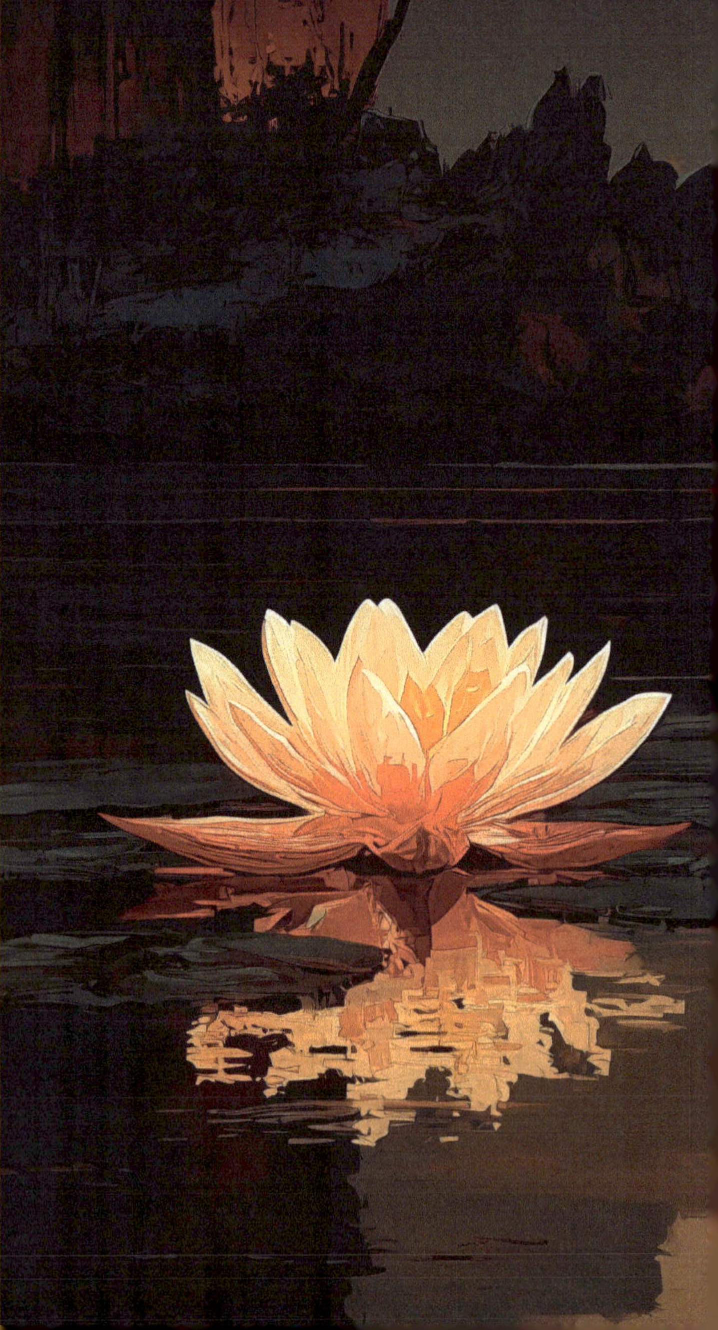

Dr. Kamal Polite, DCEM, DOM, AP, CHE, is a physician and educator with over thirty years of experience in Chinese Medicine and integrative clinical practice. His work focuses on laboratory interpretation, physiological timing, and the clinical application of ancient medical frameworks within modern healthcare settings.

Dr. Polite's training took place in both Western clinical environments and Chinese Medicine hospital systems, most notably at Yuhuangding Hospital in Yantai, Shandong, where time-based diagnostic and treatment principles were applied as practical clinical method within a modern hospital setting. That experience formed the foundation of an approach that has guided his practice ever since — one in which Western laboratory precision and Chinese Medicine pattern recognition are not two systems in conversation, but one integrated clinical method.

Over the course of his career, Dr. Polite has worked closely with individuals and families who continue to experience symptoms despite laboratory results that return within normal range. His approach helps patients understand not only what their blood tests show, but when they were drawn, what the body was doing at that moment, and what the numbers cannot capture on their own. He does not ask which system is right. He asks what the complete picture requires.

His teaching and writing are grounded in a commitment to helping people feel seen, heard, and capable of participating meaningfully in their own care. He has spent thirty years demonstrating, one patient at a time, that the missing half of most blood test interpretations is not more data — it is more context.

THANK YOU

For Reading

If you would like to learn more about having
your blood tests reviewed
with Dr. Kamal Polite through his
private practice, you may do so by
scanning the QR code below.

www.ingramcontent.com/pod-product-compliance
Lightning Source LLC
LaVergne TN
LVHW052114210926
848482LV00025B/584

* 9 7 9 8 9 9 4 7 5 0 6 1 2 *